Vacuum Extraction in Modern Obstetric Practice

Vacuum Extraction in Modern Obstetric Practice

John Patrick O'Grady, MD
Professor of Obstetrics and Gynecology,
Tufts University School of Medicine,
Director of Obstetrical Services
and Chief of the Division of Maternal-Fetal Medicine,
Baystate Medical Center, Springfield, Massachusetts, USA

Martin L. Gimovsky, MD
Associate Professor of Obstetrics and Gynecology,
Tufts University School of Medicine,
Associate Chairman of the Department of Obstetrics and Gynecology
and Director of Resident Education, Baystate Medical Center,
Springfield, Massachusetts, USA

Cyril J. McIlhargie, JD
Attorney at Law,
Chicago, Illinois, USA

The Parthenon Publishing Group
International Publishers in Medicine, Science & Technology

Published in the UK and Europe by
The Parthenon Publishing Group Limited
Casterton Hall, Carnforth,
Lancs. LA6 2LA, England

Published in the USA by
The Parthenon Publishing Group Inc.
One Blue Hill Plaza
PO Box 1564, Pearl River,
New York 10965, USA

Library of Congress Cataloging-in-Publication Data

O'Grady, John Patrick, 1945–
    Vacuum extraction in modern obstetric practice/by John Patrick O'Grady,
Martin L. Gimovsky, Cyril J. McIlhargie.
        p.   cm.
    Includes bibliographical references and index.
    ISBN 1-85070-665-4
    1. Obstetrical extraction.   I. Gimovsky, Martin L.
II. McIlhargie, Cyril J.   III. Title.
    [DNLM: 1. Vacuum Extraction Obstetrical.   WQ 415 035v 1995]
RG741.034   1995
618.8'2--dc20
DNLM/DLC
for Library of Congress   94-49184
                                                                        CIP

British Library Cataloguing in Publication Data

O'Grady, John Patrick
    Vacuum Extraction in Modern Obstetric Practice
    I. Title
    618.82
    ISBN 1-85070-665-4

Typeset by H&H Graphics, Blackburn, Lancashire
Printed in England by Bookcraft (Bath) Ltd., Midsomer Norton

Contents

Authors

SENIOR AUTHOR:

John Patrick O'Grady, MD
Professor: Obstetrics and Gynecology
Tufts University School of Medicine
Director: Obstetrical Services
Chief: Division of Maternal–Fetal Medicine
Baystate Medical Center
Springfield, Massachusetts, USA

ASSOCIATE AUTHORS:

Martin L. Gimovsky, MD
Associate Professor: Obstetrics and Gynecology
Tufts University School of Medicine
Associate Chairman: Department of Obstetrics and Gynecology
Director: Resident Education
Baystate Medical Center
Springfield, Massachusetts, USA

Cyril J. McIlhargie, JD
Attorney at Law
Chicago, Illinois, USA

Preface

Obstetric practice continues to change, particularly with regard to instrumental delivery. A rethinking of techniques for operative vaginal delivery has occurred. The complex forceps operations of a prior generation are now performed infrequently even by highly experienced practitioners. Vacuum extraction has become an increasingly popular delivery technique. Contemporary studies validate the safety of vacuum extraction and establish its utility in many procedures classically performed by forceps. The recent success of vacuum extraction is reflected in the fact that many newly graduated obstetric practitioners perform only a limited number of low or outlet forceps operations, and depend on vacuum extraction for most of their more challenging instrumental deliveries. Accompanying this accelerated interest are reports of new vacuum instruments and their successful clinical use.

Despite the similarities between vacuum extraction and forceps operations, skill in the use of forceps does not guarantee similar expertise in vacuum extraction. Specialized training is essential. Nonetheless, the major issues concerning vacuum extraction are the same as those encountered with forceps operations: case selection; evaluation of feto-pelvic proportions; accurate assessment of position/station; correct instrument placement; and the judicious application of force. To assure the safety of all types of instrumental delivery including vacuum extraction the surgeon's basic approach must be characterized by a willingness to abandon any operation which does not proceed easily.

There are some disturbing trends accompanying this accelerated interest in vacuum-assisted instrumental delivery. Deficiencies exist in obstetric training. Most residency education and continuing medical education programs do not prepare students adequately in traditional assisted delivery techniques, let alone in modern vacuum extraction operations. Also, the bulk of the available educational material concerning vacuum extraction is written by authors working in other medical systems and does not reflect practice within the United States.

Instrumentally assisted delivery remains one of the central skills of the accoucheur. In these operations, proper training, careful clinical judgement, and experience are central to safety and success. Despite changes in obstetric management that have and will affect both the type and frequency of instrumental delivery, and while the popularity of specific techniques will vary, some assistance in vaginal delivery will always be required. Regardless of the instrument or technique, the risks and benefits associated with any management decision – whether it is a forceps or vacuum extraction operation or a Cesarean delivery – must be thoroughly understood by obstetric practitioners.

For these reasons, we believe there is a need for new educational materials concerning all aspects of instrumental delivery including vacuum extraction. This has led us to prepare this clinically oriented monograph, including what we believe to be reasonable and appropriate guidelines for vacuum extraction delivery in American obstetric practice. Reflecting the realities of modern practice, the text includes a discussion of the risks and benefits of instrumental vaginal delivery and a brief review of pertinent legal issues. We trust that this book will assist clinicians in developing their skills in vacuum-assisted delivery and will contribute to the improvement of obstetric care.

John Patrick O'Grady, MD

Martin Gimovsky, MD
Cyril McIlhargie, JD

1995

DEDICATION

for

Caitlin, Cristin, Sean, and Ryan
My special deliveries

JPOG

for

Arlene, Alexis, and Matt
Winning the human race

MLG

for

Professor James W. McElharey
My friend, teacher and mentor,
who encouraged me to believe that
law could be a decent and noble profession.

Philip H. Corboy, Thomas A. Demetrio, and Marshall I. Nurenberg who
taught me much by example and encouragement.

CJM

Acknowledgements

A number of individuals assisted in the preparation of this text and we are pleased to acknowledge their contributions. The exertions of Michelle Diamond, our research assistant and office editor, were instrumental in the successful completion of this project and the importance of her assistance is especially noted. Kris Napier reviewed and critiqued the entire text, suggesting many appropriate corrections. Joyce Lavery skillfully prepared the illustrations, cheerfully agreeing to multiple changes. The secretarial assistance of Joan Kearns and Philip Zaia are also gratefully acknowledged. Finally, we applaud the support and encouragement of our spouses, friends, and colleagues during the preparation of this manuscript.

JPOG
MLG
CJM

I

The history of the vacuum extractor

The instrument is now nearly perfect . . . I fixed a small tractor to the palm of my hand and lifted up with it an iron weight of 26 pounds. I took (Dr Margulies) and others . . . to see a baddish case and fixed the tractor on.

The operation was successful. The Russian danced with joy, crying, 'C'est superb, superb, c'est immortalité à vous'.

James Young Simpson, MD (1811–1870)
Private letter, December, 1848[1]

La distance n'y fait rien; il n'y a que le premier pas qui côute.
(The distance is nothing; it is only the first step that counts.)

Marquise Du Deffand (1697–1780)
Private letter, 7 July, 1763[2]

I.1 CUPPING AND THE MEDICAL USE OF VACUUM

Vacuum-assisted delivery was born of the practice of 'cupping', the ancient therapeutic technique whereby a heated metal or glass cup or globe is applied to a lesion or skin puncture[3]. As the cup cools, a vacuum develops. This creates suction, which extracts blood or other fluids. While cupping predates Hippocrates, special surgical applications were not reported until the 17th century when cupping was used to treat depressed skull fractures and to assist at obstetric delivery[4,5].

Over nearly three centuries, increased understanding of vacuum principles exemplified by cupping were accompanied by a series of technical advances and relentless experimentation. This eventually led to the development of the modern obstetric vacuum extractor.

Historical documentation of the earliest use of a vacuum device to assist delivery is lost. However, there is reason to believe that vacuum

1

extraction for obstetric indications was practiced well before the brief mid-19th century popularity evoked by the experiments of James Simpson and others[6-8].

In November 1705, James Younge (1646–1721), an English surgeon, recorded in his case notes an instance of prolonged labor where a vacuum device was successfully applied[8,9]. It is likely that several physicians including Younge (1694), Saeman (1796), and others had developed successful vacuum delivery techniques prior to the 19th century, but either concealed this knowledge as a proprietary trade secret or at least failed to publicize their successes[7]. Nothing is known of these instruments and they did not influence later developments.

I.2 THE FIRST STEPS: J. Y. SIMPSON

The history of vacuum extraction is replete with tales of innovative individuals. Some of them invented vacuum devices, while others speculated about vacuum technique and how the physics of vacuum could be applied to surgery. Neil Arnett (1788–1874) was among the latter. In a book entitled *Elements of Physics,* Arnett[10] advocated the use of an air or 'pneumatic tractor' to assist delivery. The vacuum principle was discussed with reference to several practical demonstrations of the force required to separate evacuated globes or hemispheres. What Arnett proposed was application of vacuum technique to 'purposes of surgery', including accouchement. Arnett had a reputation as both an inventor and as an observer of nature. Among other innovations, he invented a water bed and a type of smokeless fire grate[11]. While Arnett's ideas for the medical uses of vacuum are of considerable interest, the critical comments of the 1831 Philadelphia edition's annotator, a Dr Isaac Hayes EM, MD, etc. (*sic*) demonstrate remarkable foresight. Dr Hayes disliked Arnett's proposal that a vacuum device was desirable as it could be used by those unable to apply forceps correctly. Hayes pointed out '. . . if a person deficient in dexterity could succeed in applying the (vacuum) tractor . . . it is quite probable that he would produce (as much) injury as benefit . . .'. He described how misapplication of the ventouse to the child's head or inadvertently to maternal tissues might cause damage. He also discussed how the vacuum operation might fail because of incorrect application of force, assuming the fetal scalp was successfully grasped. These arguments, with some refinement, are the same technical concerns voiced about modern vacuum-assisted instrumental deliveries.

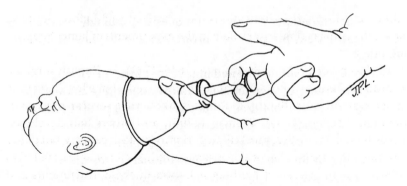

Figure I.1 Simpson's 'air tractor' vacuum extractor (1849). Redrawn from Chalmers (1971)[8]

Practical application of the vacuum principle as proposed by Arnett encountered technical difficulties. While classic techniques for cupping did produce considerable negative pressure, these methods demanded a tight seal to the patient's skin. The successful obstetric use of the vacuum principle required the development of an instrument capable of maintaining a firm grip on the fetal scalp, combined with a means for continuously regenerating the vacuum on demand due to the inevitable imperfections of the seal. In classic 'cupping', a glass or metal cup was heated with an open flame before application. Unfortunately, this provided only a single application. For obstetric use the practical problems inherent in introducing a heated cup into the vagina presented other difficulties! This was not a feasible method and other approaches had to be sought.

There were no published reports concerning vacuum extraction as a successful obstetric delivery technique until James Young Simpson announced the development of his 'suction tractor' in 1849[8,11-14] (Figure I.1). Drawing from the ideas of his predecessors, observations from nature, and his own experience, Dr Simpson invented, tested, and perfected a successful vacuum-operated device for obstetric use[11,13]. Due to Simpson's prestige and his enthusiastic medical journal report of the successful use of his 'tractor', he is regarded as the inventor of the first *practical* obstetric vacuum extractor[1,11,14,15].

Beyond technical advances of the mid-19th century, Simpson profited from the optimism and quest for innovation characteristic of this new industrial era. There was ready public and professional acceptance of experimentation and a willingness among practitioners to both publicize

3

and consider the adoption of new techniques. Refreshingly, concealment of medical devices for personal profit was at that time considered unethical.

Simpson was an influential and innovative physician. His importance in the early history of vacuum extraction is often overshadowed by his fame as the discoverer of the anesthetic properties of chloroform and his invention of a 'classic' type of obstetric forceps[7,14,15]. His championing of vacuum delivery guaranteed a serious review for both the instrument and the technique by the major obstetric practitioners of the time.

Simpson constructed his vacuum extractor from a metal vaginal speculum fitted with a suction piston. When the piston was evacuated, vacuum was produced, securing the instrument to the fetal scalp. Traction was then simply applied to the vacuum cylinder by the surgeon.

Considering the design of his 'tractor', some applications, especially to deflexed or posterior heads, must have been difficult. The instrument was long and cup positioning was restricted by the handle and pump mechanism. The same limitations are still incorporated in the design of the most modern soft cup extractors. The problem of maintaining a tight vacuum seal was also a distinct limitation. As the syringe was permanently attached to the suction cup it was not possible to continuously replenish the vacuum.

Given these problems, the forceps available to Simpson and his contemporaries were, in comparison, superior instruments. It is not surprising that professional interest in vacuum extraction soon waned. The success of vacuum-based delivery instruments would await the solution of these and other technical problems.

Despite the publicity concerning Simpson's tractor and the interest of other contemporary practitioners Simpson did not further develop his vacuum device. Thus, after the mid-19th century, vacuum extraction disappeared from the mainstream of obstetric interest for nearly 100 years.

I.3   THE INNOVATORS

Despite the lack of widespread interest in vacuum devices in the waning years of the 19th century, vacuum-operated delivery instruments continued to be described in the medical literature by a number of medical inventors including Soubhy Saleh (1857), Herbert L. Stillman (1875), and P. McCahey (1890)[8,6,16]. These devices varied widely in practicality and success.

4

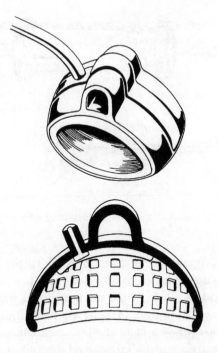

Figure I.2 Turpin's soft cup vacuum extractor (1937). Note the unusual clam shell design and the indentations near the vacuum port designed for the operator to use for finger traction

Before the introduction of the ultimately successful Malmström device, various vacuum delivery instruments were described early in the 20th century by A. D. Gladish (1933), P. Cornu (1934), R. Torpin (1937), J.S. Price (1938), M. A. Castallo (1955), Y. Couzigou (1947), W. D. Cunningham (1948), P. Körber (1950), O. Koller (1950), T. Hasegawa/R. Shiojina (1951), V. Finderle (1952), and A. G. Vincent/J. A. de Montauge (1953). While none of these devices became popular, they collectively tested, more or less successfully, all the design features that would eventually be combined in the commercially successful instruments seen today[6,8,15–17].

Technical details of several of these instruments warrant review. In 1937, R. Turpin obtained a patent on a suction delivery device, utilizing a rubber cup, that was reported to have been successfully applied in 13 cases of second stage delay[8]. Traction was applied to this device by a finger ring at the top of the cup (Figure I.2).

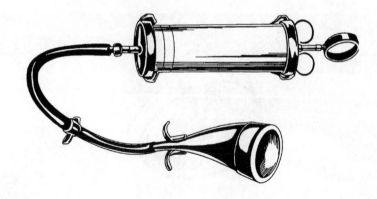

Figure I.3   Finderle vacuum extractor with evacuating syringe (1952)[17]

A review of the original patent documents for Turpin's device note a number of features common to modern designs. These include the use of a suction port independent of the traction site as well as a soft cup design. The cup was designed to close or fold upon itself, like a contraceptive diaphragm or a clam shell, to facilitate passage into the vagina. Once the instrument was introduced through the introitus, the cup resumed its proper shape, ready for cranial application. Despite these unique features, this device was never commercially successful.

Another clinically successful ventouse demonstrated before the invention of the Malmström instrument was a device developed by V. Finderle in the early 1950s[17] (Figure I.3). This extractor used an elongated metal cup of an unusual horn shape, cuffed by a flexible rubber cuff and fitted with a stopcock. Vacuum was provided by a large syringe. By 1961 Finderle reported successful applications in 212 deliveries[6,8]. Despite these clinical successes, Finderle's apparatus never achieved popularity in the West but a strikingly similar device remains in clinical use in China.

Surprisingly, *external* vacuum applications to expedite delivery experienced a brief flurry of commercial success in the early 1960s when the Emerson 'Birtheez' was introduced. This unique instrument included an abdominal dome with a vacuum pump that the mother triggered during contractions. The device created negative pressure over the abdomen while the uterus was contracting (Figure I.4).

The theory behind the Emerson and similar devices was that altering the muscular resistance of the mother's abdominal wall during uterine contractions improved fetal oxygenation, probably by decreasing

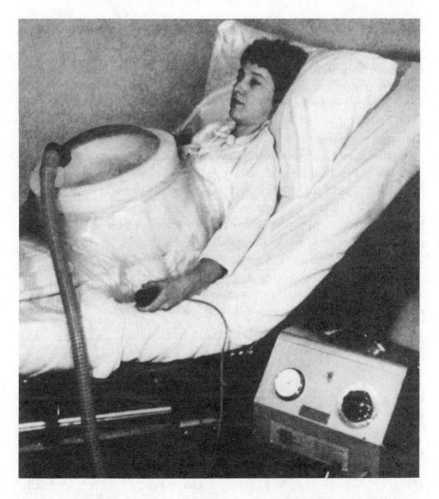

Figure I.4 Emerson 'Birtheez' extra-abdominal vacuum decompression device (1957). See text for details[18]. (Courtesy of James Edmonson, PhD, The Dittrick Museum of Medical History, Historical Division/Cleveland Health Science Library, Cleveland, OH)

intrauterine pressure. The Birtheez was also claimed to ease the pain and accelerate the speed of labor. Unfortunately, there is no evidence for a beneficial effect of abdominal decompression in otherwise normal pregnancy/labor[18]. Nonetheless, some promising results were reported in various complications of pregnancy. Samples of this fascinating device survive today only as curiosities in medical museums.

I.4 THE MALMSTRÖM EXTRACTOR

The device that repopularized vacuum extraction was the rigid cup extractor invented by T. Malmström[7,12,19]. Malmström's device and its modifications incorporated several features developed by his predecessors[20,21]. The vacuum cup contained an internal protective disc, as originally suggested by Simpson in 1849. This was designed to prevent drawing the fetal scalp into the suction port. The cup was connected by rubber tubing to a vacuum source, thus separating the pump mechanism from the cup, solving several of the application problems inherent in the original Simpson instrument. A glass collecting-bottle was positioned between the cup and the vacuum source, preventing aspiration of fluids into the vacuum pump mechanism. This was similar to the design previously suggested by McCahey and others. Finally, the Malmström system incorporated a pressure gauge, permitting the surgeon to adjust vacuum strength, so assuring a consistent application of suction force and potentially reducing the risks of scalp injury (see Chapter III, Vacuum extraction operations, Section 3.0, Traction).

Part of the original intention behind Malmström's instrument was to assist dysfunctional labors, with the theory that cervical pressure or 'irritation' stimulated uterine activity[22,23]. The procedure consisted of firm application of the fetal head against the cervix during the first stage of labor. This technique had earlier been practiced with some success by Willett[24] and Koller[8].

At present, the use of a vacuum extractor through an undilated cervix is *not* a part of accepted practice. Similarly, the 'irritation' concept of chronic cervical stimulation to treat uterine inertia has few modern adherents. Nonetheless, the Malmström vacuum extractor became rapidly popular because of its ability to function as a substitute for forceps. Applied as a traction device at full dilation and used for indications similar to those classically ascribed to forceps, Malmström's extractor rapidly proved its capability in shortening the second stage of labor by augmenting the natural forces of labor.

Following Malmström, a number of other rigid cup vacuum extractors were described by Bird, Lovset, Party, O'Neil, Halkin, and others[7,8,19-21]. Various changes were introduced to reduce the likelihood of cup detachment, facilitate application, or better protect the fetal scalp.

Bird's modification of the Malmström cup has proven to be the most popular metal extractor in American practice. In this design, the vacuum tube is attached to a lateral suction port, independent of the traction chain or cord. O'Neil's cup, which includes modifications designed to compensate for oblique traction, has also recently been introduced into the American commercial market[21] (see Chapter II, Instruments, indications, and issues). Large numbers of metal cup extractors, predominantly of Bird's design, are in the obstetric armamentarium of clinical services and an unknown number are in active use.

The popularity of metal cup extraction in the United States has been variable. Following widespread but transient interest in the early 1960s, vacuum extraction fell from favor for nearly two decades. This was due to several reasons. The complexities and assembly requirements of the original Malmström device and the formation of the unsightly chignon made vacuum extraction unpopular. In addition, several reports of serious scalp injuries appeared in the literature soon after the introduction of the instrument into American practice. As a result, the more familiar forceps delivery appeared safer to most practitioners, and interest in vacuum extraction waned until the 1980s.

I.5 RECENT DEVELOPMENTS

The pivotal modern innovation in vacuum extractor development was the introduction of new soft cup designs by Kobayashi (Dow-Corning), Wood, and others (Figures II.2–II.6)[7,19,25–27]. The introduction of low-cost, flexible plastic and improved metal suction cups, coupled with changes in physician attitude concerning assisted delivery, have contributed to a renewed popularity and supported the commercial success of vacuum extraction. Renewed interest and the development of new designs have contributed to a better understanding of vacuum technique, improving success and safety.

Experimentation with unusual vacuum traction devices has not ceased. Elliot has recently introduced an instrument consisting of a rubber or plastic 'bonnet', without a suction or vacuum port. It is designed to be unrolled or fitted onto the fetal head like an inverted parachute. Tension on the handle flattens the membrane around the fetal cranium, providing the force necessary to assist parturition (Figure I.5)[28]. The concept of inserting a net or bag to grasp the fetal head is certainly not new, as surprisingly similar examples have appeared fleetingly in the obstetric literature over the preceding two centuries. Whether such newly reinvented devices will prove any more successful than their predecessors remains to be seen.

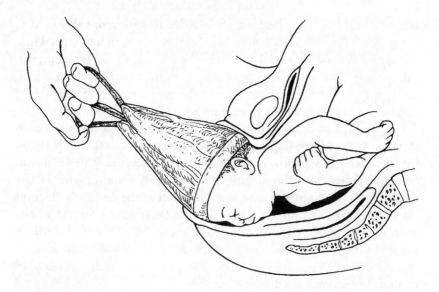

Figure I.5 Elliot's obstetric bonnet (1992). Reproduced with permission from reference[28]

In considering Elliot's reinvented cranial traction device and other new delivery instruments, an observation by Simpson in 1849 is pertinent[29]. He foresaw that '. . . if ingenuity could suggest any form of tractor which, umbrella-like, could be folded into little space for introduction, and afterwards expanded over the scalp, and then exhausted by the attached piston, it might supersede the forceps in many cases . . .'. To some extent, the application of modern technology to vacuum cup technique and design have answered Simpson's 145-year-old plea!

REFERENCES

1.   Chalmers, J.A. (1963). James Young Simpson and the 'suction-tractor'. *J. Obstet. Gynaecol. Br. Commonw.*, **70**, 94–100

2.   Du Deffand, Marquise (1763). Letter to d'Alembert, 7 July. In *The Oxford University Dictionary of Quotations*, 3rd edn., 1959, p. 198. (London: Oxford University Press)

3.   Thiery, M. (1985). Obstetric vacuum extraction. *Obstet. Gynecol. Annu.*, **14**, 73–111

4.   Hildanus (1632). *Guilhelmi Fabricii Hildani Opera*. (Frankfurt-am-Main)

5.   Johnson, T. (1665). *The Workes of That Famous Chirurgion A. Parey*, p. 243. (London)

6. Sjostedt, J.E. (1967). The vacuum extractor and forceps in obstetrics: a clinical study. *Acta Obstet. Gynecol. Scand.*, **46**, 3–208

7. O'Grady, J.P. (1988). *Modern Instrumental Delivery.* (Baltimore: Williams & Wilkins)

8. Chalmers, J.A. (1971). *The Ventouse: The Obstetric Vacuum Extractor.* (Chicago: Yearbook)

9. Younge, J. (1706–1707). An account of balls of hair taken from the uterus and ovaria of several women. *Philos. Trans. R. Soc. Lond.*, **25**, 2387

10. Arnett, N. (1831). *Elements of Physics or Natural Philosophy, General and Medical, Explained Independently of Technical Mathematics and Containing New Disquisitions and Practical Suggestions,* 2nd edn. (Philadelphia: Carney and Lea)

11. Eustace, D.L.S. (1993). James Young Simpson: the controversy surrounding the presentation of his Air Tractor (1848–1849). *J. R. Soc. Med.*, **86**, 660–3.

12. Malmström, T. (1957). The vacuum extractor. An obstetrical instrument and the parturiometer, a tokographic device. *Acta. Obstet. Gynecol. Scand.*, **36**, 7–87.

13. Simpson, J.R. (1849). On suction tractor or new mechanical power as a substitute for forceps in tedious labors. *Edinburgh Monthly J. Med. Sci.*, **32**, 556–8

14. Duns, J. (1873). *A Memoir of Sir James Y. Simpson,* pp. 288–9. (Edinburgh: Edmonston & Douglas)

15. Coues, W.P. and Simpson, W.J.Y. (1928). The prince of obstetricians. *N. Engl. J. Med.*, **199**, 221–4

16. Bret, A.J. and Coiffard, P. (1961) Les ancetrês des ventouses obstétricales. *Rev. Fr. Gynécol. d'Obstét.*, **56**, 535–53

17. Finderle, V. (1955). Extractor instead of forceps. *Am. J. Obstet. Gynecol.*, **69**, 1148–53

18. Hofmeyr, G.J. (1989). Abdominal decompression during pregnancy. In Chalmers, I., Eukin, M. and Keirse, M.J.N.C. (eds.) *Effective Care in Pregnancy and Childbirth,* pp. 647–53. (Oxford: Oxford University Press)

19. Vacca, A. (1992). *Handbook of Vacuum Extraction in Obstetric Practice.* (London: Edward Arnold)

20. Bird, G.C. (1969). Modification of Malmström's vacuum extractor. *Br. Med. J.*, **3**, 526

21. O'Neil, A.G.B., Skull, E. and Michael, C. (1981). A new method of traction for the vacuum cup. *Aust. NZ J. Obstet. Gynaecol.*, **21**, 24–5

22. Barclay, C. and Fraser, R. (1988). The history of the use of vacuum extraction. *Med. Health. Vis. Comm. Nurse*, **24**, 328–31

23. Snoeck, J. (1960). The vacuum extractor (ventouse) – an alternative to the obstetric forceps. *Proc. Roy. Soc. Med.*, **53**, 749–56

24. Willett, J.A. (1925). The treatment of placental previa by continuous weight traction – a report of seven cases. *Proc. R. Soc. Med.*, **18**, 90–4

25. Wood, J.F. (1969). An evaluation of a new plastic disposable vacuum extractor cup. *J. Am. Osteopath. Assoc.*, **66**, 1251–4

26. Laufe, L.E. and Berkus, M.D. (1992). *Assisted Vaginal Delivery*. (New York: McGraw-Hill Inc.)

27. Paul, R.H., Staisch, K.J. and Pine, S.N. (1973). The 'new' vacuum extractor. *Obstet. Gynecol.*, **41**, 800–2

28. Elliot, B.D., Ridgway, L.E., Berkus, M.D., Newton, E.R. and Peairs, W. (1992). The development and testing of new instruments for operative vaginal delivery. *Am. J. Obstet. Gynecol.*, **167**, 1121–4

29. Priestly, W.O. and Storer, H.R. (1855). *The Obstetric Memoirs and Contributions of James Y Simpson, MD FRSE*, vol. 1, pp. 498–505. (Edinburgh: Adam & Charles Black)

II

Instruments, indications, and issues

---

*It requires the greatest judgement in laborious cases when the head presents
to distinguish how long to wait, and when to assist, as well as after what
manner . . .*

William Smellie (1697–1763)
Letter to a pupil, 1749[1]

*I am very far from wishing to be understood, that I advocate the
indiscriminate interference of art . . . I wish merely to insist, that nature is
not competent to all exigencies . . . when she is permitted to proceed without
interruption . . . the sufferings of the patient might have been . . . much
abridged, by the judicious interposition of skill. Of this, from long experience,
I am entirely convinced.*

William P. Dewees (1768–1841)
A Compendius System of Midwifery, 1826[2]

II.1 EQUIPMENT

1.1 Vacuum extractor cups

Vacuum extractors currently in use in the United States are either of rigid
or flexible cup design. Rigid cup instruments include the original metal
cups of Malmström and the designs of Bird, O'Neil, and others. (Figure
II.1)[3-7]. Soft cup instruments include the cone-shaped silastic cone
(Kobayashi device) (Figure II.2) and other disposable polyethylene or
combined polyethylene–silastic cup designs, including the Neward
Enterprises, Inc. (Mityvac™) Regular and Lined Extractor Cup models,
various Columbia Medical & Surgical, Inc. (CMI) cups including the
Tender Touch™ and Tender Touch Ultra™ cup models, and the Ameda/
Egnell Silc™ Cup (Figures II.3, II.4, II.5). Also available are special design

(A)

(B)

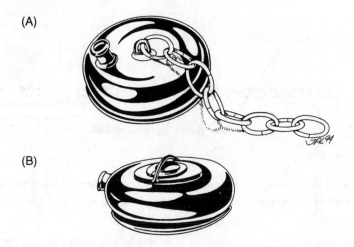

Figure II.1 (A) Bird's rigid metal vacuum extractor cup. Note the eccentrically located vacuum port and the separate, permanently affixed traction chain. The regular model is illustrated. (B) O'Neil rigid cup design. Note the rotating central cuff and the arching traction bar. The occiput posterior (OP) model of this cup is illustrated. The laterally located vacuum port facilitates application to posteriorly positioned heads. For the O'Neil cup, a separate traction handle and cord (not depicted) are attached before the cup is applied. This cup is available in 55 mm and 50 mm sizes in both anterior and posterior cup designs from Columbia Medical & Surgical, Inc., Redmond, OR., see Table II.1

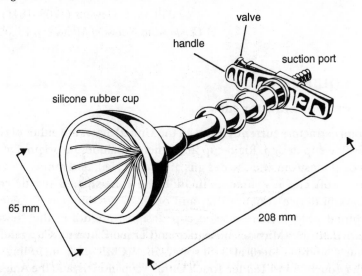

Figure II.2 Kobayashi silastic obstetric vacuum cup (Dow Corning Corporation)

14

(A)

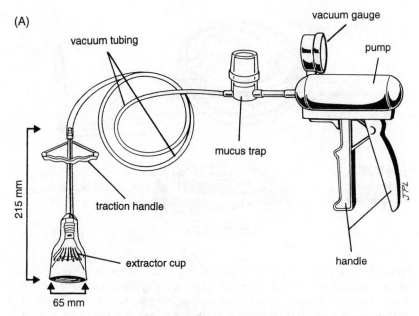

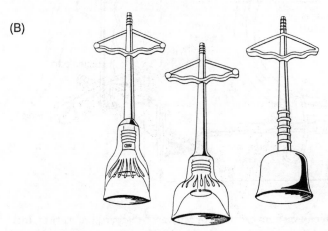

Figure II.3A Soft cup vacuum extractor, Tender Touch™ Cup (model No. 404TT) (Columbia Medical & Surgical, Inc., Redmond, OR). The extractor cup, the hand vacuum pump (model No. 001c), connecting tubing, and vacuum trap are depicted. A similar, autoclavable pump is also available from the manufacturer (model No. 101A)

(B)

Figure II.3B Soft cup vacuum extractors (Columbia Medical & Surgical, Inc., Redmond, OR). This illustrates the available cup types (left to right): Tender Touch™ Cup (60 mm model No. 404TT; 65 mm model No. 404TTL), Tender Touch Ultra™ Cup (60 mm model No. 303TT, 65 mm model No. 303TTL), and Soft Touch™ Cup (004C)

(C)

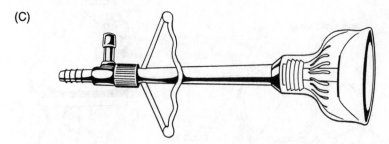

Figure II.3C Soft cup vacuum extractor: a 65 mm Tender Touch Ultra™ Cup with handle vacuum release valve (model No. 505TTL) (Columbia Medical & Surgical, Inc., Redmond, OR). See text for additional discussion and refer to Table II.1

(A)

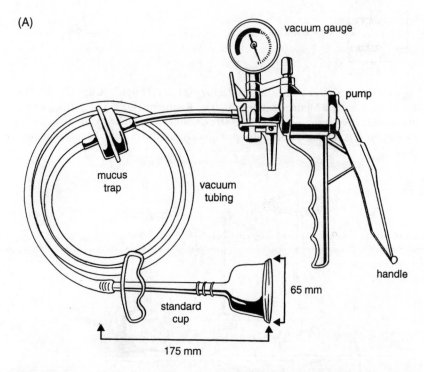

Figure II.4A Soft cup vacuum extractor by Mityvac™ (Neward Enterprises, Inc., Rancho Cucamonga, CA). This depicts the standard hand vacuum pump (model No. 001L), connecting tubing and vacuum trap with an attached standard extractor cup (model No. 004M). A regular pump with a minigrip handle (model No. 011L), an autoclavable pump (model No. 002L), and an autoclavable minigrip pump (model No. 022L) are also available from the manufacturer (see Table II.1)

(B)

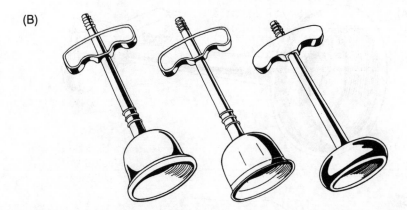

Figure II.4B Soft cup vacuum extractors (Neward Enterprises, Inc., Rancho Cucomongo, CA). This illustrates the three available Mityvac cup types: (left to right): Lined Cup™ (model No. 010M), Standard™ Cup (model No. 004M), and 'M' Style™ Mechanical Pull Vacuum Extractor Cup (model No. 007M)

(C)

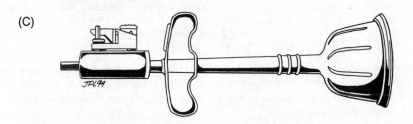

Figure II.4C Soft cup vacuum extractors (Neward Enterprises, Inc., Rancho Cucomongo, CA). A lined cup model similar to model No. 010M above with a vacuum release valve positioned at the cup handle is also now available (refer to Table II.1)

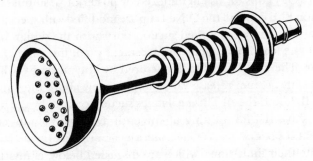

Figure II.5 Soft cup vacuum extractor cup (Silc™ Cup) (Ameda/Egnell, Inc., Cary, Il)

17

(A)

(B)

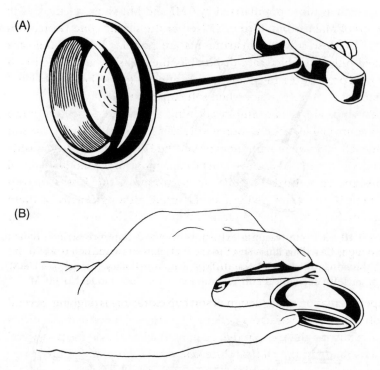

Figure II.6 (A) Mityvac 'M' Style™ Mechanical Pull Vacuum Extractor Cup design (model No. 007M, Neward Enterprises, Inc., Rancho Cucamongo, CA). (B) This depicts the flexibility possible at the cup/handle junction, improving the application to deflexed heads

plastic and metal cups, such as the Mityvac 'M' Style™ Mechanical Pull Vacuum Extractor Cup (Figure II.6) and the Bird[8] and O'Neil[9] occiput posterior (OP) cups for use in deflexed or posterior positions. The New Generation Bird cup and the O'Neil cup are modified with special traction systems and laterally positioned suction ports with the design intention to reduce the likelihood of cup displacement when the force of traction is oblique. The cup designs manufactured by Mityvac and CMI are also available with vacuum release valves immediately above the cup handle (Figures II.3c and II.4c). This facilatates suction control by the operator. Refer to Table II.1 for a listing of currently available vacuum cups and equipment suppliers.

Despite their limitations, which are discussed below, many clinicians now favor disposable polyethylene or polyethylene/silastic soft cup designs, such as those popularized by CMI and Mityvac, over the classic rigid cups of Malmström, Bird or O'Neil or the silastic cone (Kobayashi device)[6,11]. These soft cup instruments are popular because they are packaged fully assembled, are disposable, inexpensive, and effective in most outlet procedures. In addition, there appears to be a lower associated incidence of fetal scalp injury when soft cups are used[12-15].

These cups are usually employed using a hand-held vacuum pump but any controllable vacuum source will suffice (e.g. wall suction, suction machine, etc.). Some practitioners prefer the Dow Corning (Kobayashi) extractor, the original Malmström metal cup, or one of the modified metal cup designs (e.g. Bird, O'Neil). Unfortunately, the Dow Corning instrument is no longer being manufactured, although many of these instruments are still in clinical service. While the rigid cups are currently less popular, the bulk of the published literature on vacuum extraction experience is based on the use of these instruments and they remain the instruments of choice for certain vacuum extraction operations as is discussed later in the text.

Experimentation in the design of soft cup extractors is ongoing. Several new soft cup plastic extractors designed by the two major manufacturers (CMI and Mityvac) have entered the commercial market in the last several years. Less happily, the clinical differences between many of these new instruments is inconsequential. This recent proliferation of models is unencumbered by evidence attesting to any specific benefit from each unique design (Table II.1).

1.2 Comparisons between instruments

While new vacuum cup designs have entered the market rapidly, there are limited clinical studies which assess their performance in comparison to more conventional instruments. This scarcity of comparative studies is not surprising. Clinical investigations of vacuum extractors are difficult to conduct both because of the expense and due to the many variables affecting study results which are unrelated to the design of an individual cup. Case selection, the strength of the vacuum used, cup placement, traction technique, fetal head position, and operator skill all influence both extraction success and safety.

Clinicians are cautioned that the common manufacturer's claims of reduced fetal or maternal risk for a particular instrument or modification await verification by prospective testing in carefully planned studies. While

Table II.1   American equipment suppliers: vacuum extraction devices, 1995

Device	Supplier
Rigid Cup Extractors	
Malmström Bird Cup (Regular and occiput posterior models)	Ameda/Egnell 765 Industrial Drive Cary, Illinois 60013 (708) 639-2900 (800) 323-8750 (708) 639-7895 Fax
O'Neil Cup (50 mm anterior cup, model No. VC1151; 55 mm anterior cup, model No. VC1153) (50 mm posterior occiput posterior cup, model No. VC1152 55 mm posterior occiput posterior cup, model No. VC1154)	Columbia Medical & Surgical, Inc. P.O. Box 1530 Redmond, Oregon 97756-1530 (800) 548-8667 (503) 548-7738 (503) 548-8066 Fax
Plastic Disposable Extractors	
Mityvac 'M' Style™ Mechanical Pull Vacuum Extractor Cup (model No. 007M) Mityvac Standard™ Vacuum Extractor Cup (model No. 004M) Mityvac Lined™ Vacuum Extractor Cup (model No. 010M)	Neward Enterprises, Inc. 9251 Archibald Avenue Rancho Cucamongo, CA 91730 (800) 648-9822 (714) 980-4654 Fax
Ameda/Egnell Soft Vacuum Assist Cup (Silc™ Cup)	Ameda/Egnell, Inc. 765 Industrial Drive Cary, Illinois 60013 (708) 639-2900 (800) 323-8750 (708) 639-7895 Fax
CMI Vacuum Delivery System Tender Touch™ Vacuum Extractor Cup with vacuum handle release (60 mm, model No. 404TT; 65 mm, model No. 404TTL)	Columbia Medical & Surgical, Inc. P.O. Box 1530 Redmond, Oregon 97756-1530 (503) 548-7738 (800) 548-8667 (503) 548-8066 Fax
Tender Touch Ultra™ Cup Vacuum Extractor without vacuum handle release (60 mm, model No. 303TT; 65 mm, model No. 303TTL)	Columbia Medical & Surgical, Inc. details as above

continued

Table II.1 *continued*

Device	Supplier
Tender Touch Ultra™ Cup Vacuum Extractor with vacuum handle release (60 mm, model No. 505TT; 65 mm, model No. 505TTL) Soft Touch™ Vacuum Extractor Cup (model No. 004C)	Columbia Medical & Surgical, Inc. P.O. Box 1530 Redmond, Oregon 97756-1530 (503) 548-7738 (800) 548-8667 (503) 548-8066 Fax

some relationship exists between cup design, success in extraction, and the likelihood of injury, reliable data concerning most of the newly introduced devices are either incomplete or non-existent. At present, the claims for greater safety or success for a specific new cup design should be discounted until appropriate comparative studies have been published. Commercial promotion in this field commonly exceeds clinically documented merit – a deficiency that will be remedied slowly.

In routine low or outlet extractions, design differences between the cups and differences in cup size (diameters) are clinically insignificant. In more complicated operations choice of a specific cup model is more important. Ultimately, though, minor modifications of cup design are of much less consequence than a correct anatomic application and meticulous surgical technique.

Despite limited data, some comparative observations have been published. As an example, in general, soft or flexible cups have more limited applications and may have a higher reported incidence of extraction failure. However, these cups are also associated with less cosmetic injury to the fetus than metal cup designs[12-15] (Table II.2). Disposable polyethylene extractors are a more effective outlet delivery instrument than the silastic cone (Kobayashi device)[10]. Soft cups apparently have a reduced risk of scalp injury when compared to rigid models but, by design, are limited in the traction force that can be applied and the type of applications possible. Thus, extraction failures are more common in a number of series with soft cup designs, especially in comparison to forceps or metal cups[14,16,17] (Table II.3). Reports of failure rates with the silastic cone (Kobayashi device) have been quite variable and are likely due to differences in technique and case selection[13,18,19].

Cup detachment is generally observed more frequently with the Kobayashi cone, especially at the outlet where the absence of tissue pressure permits cup deformation and resultant loss of vacuum[12].

Table II.2 Effect of soft vs. hard vacuum extractor cups on significant scalp trauma*

Study	Soft cup n (%)	Metal cup n (%)	Odds ratio (95% CI)
Cohn et al.[14†]	18/31 (14)	23/127 (18)	0.7 (0.4–1.4)
Hammarström et al.[15‡]	2/50 (4)	6/50 (12)	0.3 (0.1–1.4)
Kuit et al.[129†]	3/50 (6)	11/50 (22)	0.23 (0.06–0.87)
Chenoy and Johanson[12**]	22/101 (22)	37/98 (38)	0.46 (0.24–0.86)
Typical odds ratio (95% CI)			0.50 (0.46–0.54)

*Reprinted from reference 12 with permission; †Silc™ Cup vs. Bird & Malmström Cup; **Silc™ Cup vs. Malmström Cup; ‡Silastic cone (Kobayashi) vs. Malmström Cup; CI, confidence intervals

Table II.3 Effects of soft vs. hard vacuum extractor cups on failure to deliver with selected instrument*

Study	Soft cup n (%)	Metal cup n (%)	Odds ratio (95% CI)
Hofmeyr et al.[10***]	3/13 (23)	0/18 (–)	12.8 (1.2–99)
Cohn et al.[14†]	21/31 (16)	13/127 (10)	1.7 (0.8–3.4)
Hammarström et al.[121**]	9/50 (18)	1/50 (2)	5.8 (1.6–21)
Kuit et al.[129†]	5/50 (10)	2/50 (4)	2.7 (0.5–14)
Chenoy and Johanson[12‡]	15/101 (15)	13/98 (13)	1.14 (0.5–2.54)
Typical odds ratio (95% CI)			1.75 (1.55–2)

*Reprinted from reference 12 with permission: †Silc™ Cup vs. Bird & Malmström Cup; ‡Silc cup vs. Malmström Cup; **Silastic cone (Kobayashi) vs. Malmström Cup; ***Silc™ Cup and Silastic cone (Kobayashi) vs. New Bird and O'Neil Cup; CI, confidence intervals

II.2 OPERATIONS

2.1 Definitions

The standard definitions suggested by the American College of Obstetricians and Gynecologists (ACOG) for instrumental delivery operations include: *outlet, low,* and *mid* operations depending upon clinical examination, assessing the position and station of the fetal head at the commencement of the procedure[20-22]. When evaluated clinically, these new definitions appear to correlate with fetal–maternal risk, at least for forceps[23]. While these ACOG guidelines were originally written for forceps operations, the same descriptions may be applied to vacuum extraction operations with minor modifications.

There are three basic procedures: *outlet vacuum extraction, low vacuum extraction,* and *mid-vacuum extraction* (Table II.4). Subclassifications for vacuum operations based on cranial positioning are included but are of limited utility as rotation occurs spontaneously with successful descent. A simple distinction between occiput posterior and anterior positions is proposed in these coding suggestions. Because of frequent deflection, occiput transverse positions are included in the OP category. The definitions include special categories for vacuum extraction at Cesarean delivery and for operations not otherwise classified.

Note that station as used in this proposed classification and throughout the text follows the recent ACOG recommendations and is reported *in centimeters* (± 5)[20-22]. This reflects the clinical estimate of the distance between the leading bony portion of the fetal skull and the plane of the maternal ischial spines. In this text, when station is reported, two numbers will be provided (e.g. + 2/5 cm). The first number indicates the station as estimated by pelvic examination – plus 2 in the example given. The second number reminds the reader that the 5 cm scale for reporting station is the one intended. Clinicians will observe that *stations in this new 5-point scale do not correspond with station as classically reported on the ± 3 (or 4) scale originally taught to many obstetricians.* In reporting station in the medical record, use of a recording convention such as suggested above will help reduce confusion and permit a better comparison between the examinations recorded by various clinicians.

2.2 Indications: vacuum extraction

The indications for operative vaginal delivery are either maternal or fetal[4-6,11,20-22]. These include: a prolonged second stage of labor; indicated (and elective) shortening of the second stage; and presumed fetal jeopardy (non-reassuring fetal status on the basis of heart rate pattern or auscultatory findings, fetal distress).

Table II.4 Proposed classification for vacuum extraction procedures according to fetal station and cranial position[20–22]

Type of Operation*	Description of classification**
Outlet vacuum operation	The fetal head is at or on the perineum; the scalp is visible at the introitus without separating the labia; the fetal skull has reached the pelvic floor
Low vacuum operation	The position/station of the fetal head does not fulfill the criterion for an outlet operation; the leading edge of the fetal skull is at station $\geq + 2/5$ cm, but has not reached the pelvic floor[†]
Subdivisions	(1) Position is occiput anterior (OA, LOA, ROA) (2) Position is occiput posterior (OP, LOP, ROP) or transverse (LOT, ROT)
Mid-vacuum operation	Station $< + 2/5$ cm. The fetal head is engaged but the criterion for outlet or low operations are not fulfilled
Subdivisions:	(1) Position is occiput anterior (OA, LOA, ROA) (2) Position is occiput posterior (OP, LOP, ROP) or transverse (LOT, ROT)
Vacuum-assisted Caesarean delivery	This includes all vacuum-assisted Cesarean deliveries, unspecified technique
Special vacuum operations	This includes vacuum extraction operations not specified; full details are described in a *dictated* operative note
High vacuum operation	Such procedures are not included in the classification

*Note: formal dictation of *all* vacuum operations regardless of apparent ease is suggested (see Chapter II, Section 3.1, Documentation, for details)

**The type of operation coded is determined by pelvic examination noting the position and station of the fetal head at the time the extraction is performed

[†]Station (+ 5 to –5) is defined as the distance in cm between the leading bony portion of the fetal skull and the plane of maternal ischial spines and is recorded in the medical record as: ± 5/5 cm. See text for details

2.2.1 Prolonged second stage

Second stage labor of more than 2 h without a regional or epidural anesthetic or 3 h with such an anesthetic is considered prolonged for nulliparous women. For parous women, these time intervals become 1 and 2 h, respectively. Any instrumental assistance for the indication of a prolonged second stage demands caution[24,25]. Failure to descend normally in the second stage is an important clinical sign, suggesting the possibility of malpresentation, cranial deflection or other malpositioning, or, rarely, true fetopelvic disproportion. Non-operative management of this labor abnormality may include expectant management (i.e. a simple prolongation of labor), oxytocin stimulation, or permitting the effects of analgesia/anesthesia to subside. These and other issues are discussed in detail below (see Section 3.6, Clinical evaluation of pelvic adequacy below and Chapter IV, Complications and birth injuries, Section 2.5, Shoulder dystocia).

2.2.2 Shortening of second stage

Shortening of the second stage of labor is a *potential indication* for instrumental delivery. Possible clinical settings are mothers with cardiac, cerebrovascular, or neuromuscular conditions where voluntary expulsive efforts are either contraindicated or impossible. Additional situations might include poor second stage expulsive efforts due to maternal exhaustion, limited ability to co-operate, overly dense epidural analgesia/ anesthesia, or other clinical settings[25]. Consideration of encouragement, oxytocin administration, and maternal repositioning are advised when maternal expulsive efforts weaken in the second stage[7].

If a simple outlet or 'liftout' procedure is possible (i.e. when the fetal head is on the perineum and oriented within 45° of the anteroposterior diameter) and there is no suspicion of disproportion, the second stage may be terminated electively. Such 'prophylactic' instrumentation was part of standard American practice for many years but is now less commonly performed. This procedure is under critical re-evaluation[6,26–30]. Nonetheless, such deliveries are associated with no difference in perinatal outcome as compared to simple, spontaneous deliveries[31].

2.2.3 Presumed fetal jeopardy/fetal distress

In the case of presumed fetal jeopardy, the clinician reasonably believes there is a risk to the fetus. Other terms used include *non-reassuring fetal heart rate status* (based on auscultory findings) or *non-reassuring fetal heart rate tracing* (assuming an electronic monitor is used) or *fetal distress*. In these clinical situations, prompt evaluation is indicated and emergent delivery may be required. Fetal scalp sampling or acoustic stimulation, especially in the presence of an equivocal electronic monitor tracing, can be helpful in reaching a management decision. Underlying pathophysiology can include abruptio placentae, cord prolapse or entanglements, or other acute (and often unexplained) fetal bradycardias. Clinical evidence for fetal distress might include abnormal fetal heart rate patterns, observations of cord prolapse, sudden maternal or fetal–maternal hemorrhage, meconium passage, abnormal scalp or cord pH values, or histological abnormalities in the placenta[32,33].

Recurrent late second stage bradycardias are common especially with occiput posterior presentations. These heart rate changes are usually of minimal clinical significance, provided the fetal heart rate returns to base line, beat-to-beat variability is retained, and the decelerating patterns do not persist beyond approximately 30 min. However, fixed bradycardias or recurrent severe decelerations accompanied by prolonged loss of beat-to-beat variability can require expedited vaginal delivery if prompt spontaneous parturition does not occur. Marked cord compression and bradycardia is accompanied by a drop in fetal pH by approximately 0.02 pH units per min, providing some time for observation and the consideration of options[34]. The demand for intervention is more pressing if the fetus has begun the second stage with a low or abnormal pH.

Cord prolapse, abruptio placentae, or persisting bradycardias at high station ($\leq +1/5$ cm) even at full dilation are best managed by Cesarean delivery. In less extreme circumstances, the delivery route is dictated by station and position, the feto–pelvic relationship, and operator skill. During an attempted vaginal delivery complicated by apparent fetal distress, an experienced clinician remains at the perineum, encouraging bearing-down efforts and prepared to assist instrumentally while other personnel *simultaneously* prepare for Cesarean delivery. A Cesarean operation should be performed if spontaneous or assisted vaginal delivery is not imminent when the operative preparations have been completed. While operative heroics have no place in obstetric management, we are convinced that emergent, expedited vaginal delivery using forceps or vacuum extractor by experienced personnel is appropriate in *select* cases of presumed fetal jeopardy in a rapidly progressing labor in the setting of unquestioned pelvic adequacy[7] (see Trials of instrumental delivery,

Section 2.4 below for a full discussion of the suggested management of such acute situations).

When urgent or emergent vaginal delivery is performed, umbilical arterial and venous cord gases should be obtained and the placenta submitted for histological examination[32]. The surgeon must also document the operative indications and delivery procedures in a dictated note in the medical record. The attending physician should discuss the same details with the mother and her husband or family after the procedure if it was not possible before (see Section 3.1, Documentation below and Chapter V, Legal issues, Section 4, Documentation and Section 5, Communication).

2.3   Contraindications and special applications

Vacuum extraction is inappropriate in some clinical settings. The most important contraindication is *operator inexperience* with the instrument or *inability to achieve a proper application* due to fetal position or station. Other important contraindications are: an inadequate trial of labor; uncertainty concerning fetal position and/or station; a suspicion of fetopelvic disproportion; an inappropriately high fetal head; and malpositioning (e.g. breech, face, brow).

The vacuum extractor should be used with caution in premature infants, as the inherent risks of fetal complication (such as fetal intracranial hemorrhage) may be greater[35]. More recent experience suggests that this restriction may be unnecessarily conservative[36]. Nonetheless, *elective* vacuum operations on infants of less than 36 weeks gestation are, in general, contraindicated. The case for *indicated* procedures is less clear as data regarding safety are limited.

There is a minimal risk of fetal hemorrhage if the extractor is applied following scalp sampling or application of a spiral scalp electrode[37,38]. Such procedures are not absolute contraindications to extraction operations but do require a prudent approach to the procedure; many successful and safe extractions have been reported. The caveat is that the scalp electrode must not interfere with correct cup placement. If vacuum extraction follows scalp sampling, the use of clear vacuum tubing, which is observed periodically for the presence of bloody effluent, is advised. Evidence of marked fetal blood loss from a scalp incision, augmented by vacuum application, requires immediate assessment of fetal well-being and the termination of the extraction effort. This should be a rare event, at best.

At higher stations, vacuum extraction operations follow the same restrictions as do forceps procedures. Delivery of the second baby of a twin delivery is a partial exception. In experienced hands, the well-flexed head of the second twin can often be grasped easily soon after it negotiates the pelvic inlet and becomes engaged. Traction combined with directed maternal expulsion efforts ordinarily result in prompt delivery. Care must be taken, however, to assure correct cup application while avoiding head displacement and possible cord prolapse. Real-time ultrasound scanning provides valuable information as the second twin is positioned to enter the maternal pelvis.

In the unusual cases requiring instrumental assistance during Cesarean delivery, vacuum extraction may be used; the vectus blade (Murless or similar) or modified forceps are additional choices[6,39-41]. Instrumental assistance should always be considered but is uncommonly indicated if there is difficulty in cranial extraction, except in special circumstances. A forceps or vacuum extractor application is not the best answer in many cases of difficulty. Consideration of the clinical problem is needed to determine the best approach.

Difficulty with cranial extraction generally arises from an inadequate myometrial incision or if there has been a prolonged labor from a deeply engaged, heavily molded fetal head. The original surgical incision may be the problem. For Cesarean delivery, the abdominal wound should be approximately 15 cm long. This is the 'Allis Clamp' test – an average Allis clamp is 15 cm long. If the original incision restricts the surgeon's exposure, making the cranial extraction difficult, prompt, bilateral extension of the abdominal wound is all that is required. In selected instances the rectus muscles will also need to be incised or reflected from their insertion to provide adequate space. When the fetal head is impacted, manual intraoperative vaginal displacement (i.e. upward pressure on the fetal head from below) facilitates cranial delivery and reduces the risk of wound laceration. When the fetal head is impacted, vaginal displacement is a more certain and safer procedure than either a forceps or vacuum application. The forceps or the vacuum extractor *are* uniquely helpful in cranial extraction at Cesarean delivery when the fetal head is high or the fetus malpositioned – specifically in an oblique or transverse lie. In these situations, the instrument fixes and extracts what can be an otherwise undeliverable fetal head, avoiding the need for version and breech extraction.

2.4 Trials of instrumental delivery

There is an important distinction between *a trial of instrumental delivery* and a *failed instrumental delivery*. If close clinical evaluations of pelvis and fetus have been performed properly and cases of disproportion excluded, few instrumental deliveries will need to be conducted in the operating room with parallel preparations for Cesarean delivery. Nonetheless, an important but limited role remains for such carefully conducted trials of instrumental delivery[6,42–44].

In a trial of instrumental delivery by vacuum extraction (or forceps) the operator assesses the clinical setting and applies the instrument, having made prior preparations for Cesarean delivery if the attempt fails[6]. In a properly conducted trial *the surgeon is prepared for immediate Cesarean delivery if the proposed vaginal procedure is not successful or if an attempt at vaginal delivery is judged inappropriate after reassessment in the operating room.*

The term failed instrumental delivery, or failed vacuum extraction/ forceps delivery is reserved for cases in which *forceps or the vacuum extractor are applied with the anticipation of vaginal delivery but the procedure fails, with or without injury to the mother and fetus.* In these cases, no prior preparations for Cesarean delivery have been made. Some of these failures occur because of true disproportion, improper instrument placement, and/or traction technique (Table II.5). Most, however, result from errors in

Table II.5 Causes of vacuum extraction failure[4,5,6,11]

---

(1) Malpresentation:
    (a) cranial deflection
    (b) occiput posterior position
        asynclitism
(2) Uterine retraction or Bandl's ring
(3) Uterine constriction ring
(4) Incomplete cervical dilation
(5) Technical equipment failure:
    (a) pump dysfunction/inadequate vacuum
    (b) undiagnosed system leaks
(6) Traction failure/cup displacement:
    (a) oblique traction or incorrect force vector
    (b) traction not co-ordinated with maternal efforts
    (c) inadequate vacuum
(7) Incorrect cup application (not at cranial pivot or flexing point)
(8) Failure to recruit maternal voluntary expulsive efforts
(9) Use of obstetric anesthesia rather than analgesia
(10) True cephalo- or fetopelvic disproportion

---

clinician judgement. The failure to plan in advance for foreseeable extraction failures, not adhering to standard protocol, or not carefully limiting traction efforts, and/or failing to initiate preparations for Cesarean delivery in uncertain cases can result in serious fetal/maternal injuries and places the surgeon and the institution in an unnecessary and difficult position.

It is well to remember that clinical obstetrics is not an exact science. The exercise of judgment includes the possibility for error. All instrumental deliveries are best considered trials, as even the most experienced surgeons can experience an occasional failure. Some emphasis is appropriate. Controlling the limits of effort is critical when an instrument has been applied, especially in cases of possible disproportion and presumed fetal jeopardy/fetal distress. When prompt delivery does not occur, the clinician must resist the initial tendency to exert greater effort to achieve delivery. Unanticipated failures of instrumentation are largely due to incomplete assessment of the initial clinical situation[43,44]. *After accurate application and reasonable effort, should problems arise with an instrumental delivery, the correct response is to immediately stop and reassess*[6].

2.4.1 *Personnel and setting*

Anesthetic assistance, operating room personnel, nursing assistance, and the services of a pediatrician or other personnel trained in fetal resuscitation need to be identified and informed of the surgeon's intention *prior* to attempting a trial of instrumental delivery.

Trials of instrumental delivery are conducted in the operating room in a setting where prompt Cesarean delivery is possible if the effort at vaginal delivery is unsuccessful. There are costs involved in the use of personnel and equipment in conducting trials of instrumental delivery in the operating theater. These expenses are more than offset by the costs of *failing* to make these preparations if urgent or emergent Cesarean delivery is necessary.

2.4.2 *Anesthesia/analgesia*

Consultation with the anesthesiologist or other personnel trained in the administration of anesthesia precedes a properly conducted trial.

Obviously, vaginal operative procedures require adequate *analgesia* to offset maternal discomfort. However, the team must also be prepared to provide prompt *anesthesia* suitable for Cesarean delivery if the vaginal trial is not successful. Epidural blockade, fulfilling both demands, is usually ideal. If epidural anesthesia is not available, or if other reasons preclude its use, the vacuum trial is best conducted with pudendal blockade or with only 'local and vocal' anesthesia. If so, an extraction failure may be followed by general inhalation anesthetic or, on rare occasions, a spinal, depending upon the speed required in the delivery and the anesthesiologist's preference.

General anesthesia should not be administered in advance for a vacuum extraction trial, as the surgeon needs an awake and co-operative patient to assist in fetal expulsion. In addition, if the vaginal route proves impractical or impossible, the general anesthesia will have been present for a prolonged period of time before delivery of the child occurs, compounding the risk for neonatal depression.

The responsible practitioner must take charge of the conduct of the delivery and direct the actions of the mother and the other assistants. Beginning the effort with an openly stated, clear, and simple pronouncement outlining the procedure to be followed is prudent. A fearful or extremely agitated mother may consume her reservoir of strength and tolerance in ineffectual pushing or simply become distraught and lose focus without kind but firm direction. The clinician must command her attention, recruit her efforts, and make it clear that a plan exists and that she is expected to be an active participant.

2.4.3 Counseling

Prior to conducting a trial, the clinical situation is best discussed candidly with the mother and her family or attendants. Obviously, if the need for delivery is emergent, this may be a brief review indeed. However, in most instances, the need for instrumental assistance is suspected long before the procedure is performed. The mother and family should be informed of the attendant's concern when difficulties are identified and not simply surprised by a sudden demand for operative delivery. Unfortunately, a substantial number of patients may receive (or at least report receiving!) little information concerning the reasons for their instrumental delivery[45].

Ideally, the clinician's assessment of the reasons for poor progress are reviewed and the recommendation for an operative trial is presented to the woman and her support person(s) with a discussion of the nature, purpose, and risks of the proposed operation(s). The possible alternatives of either an abdominal or vaginal birth under the unique clinical situation present and the attendant risks of either choice are also discussed. If a vaginal trial is elected, no *assurance* of outcome is given but *reassurance* concerning the limits of effort are appropriate and advisable. In the opinion of the authors, it is appropriate, when feasible, to conduct such trials with a member of the family present in the operating room. This person supports the parturient and is privy to the various clinical discussions. If less than perfect results occur, at minimum such preparations provide a basis for better understanding and acceptance by the mother and family of what transpired within the delivery room. This approach also provides a basis for demonstrating active involvement of the family in the decision-making process. Regardless of outcome, a more complete explanation of what has transpired is provided later when mother and baby are stable.

Before the delivery, if circumstances permit, it is desirable that the clinician either write or dictate his/her intentions concerning the proposed operation. After the trial, *regardless of the outcome*, a full procedure note is dictated, indicating the clinical setting, the findings, the procedures performed or attempted, and complications encountered (see Chapter V, Legal issues, Section 4, Documentation and Section 5, Communication).

2.4.4   Conduct of the procedure

If delivery is not achieved or imminent after four traction efforts or a maximum of two cup displacements, *assuming descent began with the initial pull,* the procedure is abandoned[46] (Table II.6). If vacuum extraction efforts have failed, the forceps should not be applied except with great trepidation. If, however, it is determined that the vacuum extraction effort failed for technical reasons (malapplication, equipment failure, etc.), there is some limited justification for further additional effort with another instrument. However, it is to be strictly understood that forceps trials following a failed vacuum extraction operation, or the reverse procedure of vacuum extraction to follow forceps, *are conducted only by the most experienced of vaginal surgeons and should be considered as exceptions from the usual rules of conduct* [43,47]. The risks of fetal and maternal injury are increased in this setting[46,48].

Table II.6 Number of tractions required in vacuum extraction and forceps deliveries (see text for a full discussion)*

No. of traction efforts	Malmström vacuum extractor ($n = 433$)	Forceps** ($n = 555$)
1–2	296 (68.4%)	213 (38.4%)
3–4	108 (24.9%)	270 (48.6%)
≥ 5	29 (6.7%)	72 (12.9%)

*Neonates < 600 g excluded; other exclusions include breech presentations, Cesarean deliveries, transverse lies, and most multiple gestations. Twins were included if ≥ 600 g and one delivered spontaneously, by vertex. **Type unspecified. (Modified with permission from reference 46)

Continuous attention to fetal status, by serial fetal heart rate determinations by Doppler device or simple auscultation, or by continuous electronic monitoring, is critical in trials of instrumental delivery. In some outwardly appropriate trials, reassuring tracings before instrumentation have elicited no particular concern; therefore, the subsequent move to Cesarean delivery was urgent rather than emergent. Unfortunately, when the uterus was opened, the child was found to be in extremis or even stillborn. Presumably, the traction occasioned by the instrumental trial resulted in cord compromise (or some other unknown event), and unrecognized bradycardias occurred with eventual fetal injury.

Following an unsuccessful or a failed trial with any instrument, and regardless of the intensity of the effort employed, the best practice is to apply an internal fetal monitoring scalp clip/electrode. The fetal heart rate is thereafter continuously monitored with a standard electronic fetal monitor by observation of the paper strip and/or by listening for the beep accompanying each systole. If this is not possible, the fetal heart is auscultated immediately and then after every contraction or minimally every 5–10 min until the surgical skin preparation for the Cesarean delivery is begun. The rule is that fetal heart rate determinations in the operating room must be conducted throughout the case with the same (or increased) frequency and with similar attention to pattern as was practiced in the labor room.

If a fixed fetal bradycardia is diagnosed, the surgical assistant(s) and the anesthesiologist are instructed to proceed expeditiously with preparations for a Cesarean while the senior surgeon attempts upward vaginal displacement of the fetal head and assists in lateral recumbency positioning or wedging of the mother's hip. Oxygen is also administered to the mother. These maneuvers alone may result in a resolution of the bradycardia. Other attendants prepare for possible neonatal resuscitation. If a slow fetal heart rate continues, the surgeon then proceeds to a brief, intense scrub and re-enters the room where, usually, the final anesthesia and surgical preparations are complete. Prompt Cesarean delivery follows.

If the presenting part has descended with traction during an unsuccessful vaginal trial, or if molding was present at low station, it is prudent to station an assistant under the drapes with instructions to lift the fetal head from below during the Cesarean delivery. This greatly facilitates cranial delivery, while avoiding injury to the lower uterine segment, and does not increase the risk of postoperative infection (see Section 2.3, Contraindications and special applications above).

II.3 SPECIAL ISSUES

Issues concerning the practice of vacuum delivery discussed in this section include appropriate medical record documentation and the ongoing debate regarding the safety and efficacy of forceps vs. vacuum extraction in various clinical settings.

3.1 Documentation

Proper documentation is an essential part of the surgeon's responsibility in operative deliveries[6,20]. All operative deliveries, whether by forceps or vacuum extraction, require full documentation (Table II.7). It is the responsibility of the surgeon to record pertinent data in the medical record by a detailed hand-written note and by formal dictation of an operative report, or, preferably, by both methods.

In instances where presumed fetal jeopardy (fetal distress, non-reassuring fetal status, etc.) is the indication for operative intervention or there is an unanticipated and untoward neonatal outcome, it is prudent to obtain umbilical arterial and venous pH values and to report how the original diagnosis was established (e.g. fetal heart rate patterns, reference to the results of acoustic stimulation, and/or data from fetal scalp sampling, etc.). In these circumstances, the placenta should also be submitted for histological examination[32].

34

Table II.7   Instrumental delivery: issues in routine documentation*

1.0   Setting:

   1.1   Labor course (Partographic analysis)

   1.2   Maternal condition

   1.3   Fetal condition:
      1.3.1   EFM/auscultation patterns
      1.3.2   scalp pH
      1.3.3   response to scalp stimulation
      1.3.4   meconium presence
      1.3.5   other observations

   1.4   Informed consent process

2.0   Clinical evaluations:

   2.1   Abdominal examination:
      2.1.1   estimated fetal weight
      2.1.2   fetal lie, presentation
      2.1.3   descent/engagement by Philpott, and/or Leopold's maneuvers

   2.2   Pelvic examination:
      2.2.1   position, station, cervical dilation, membrane status
      2.2.2   cranial deflection, molding, caput, asynclitism
      2.2.3   pelvic architecture/type
      2.2.4   cranial descent/flexion with contraction and/or fundal
           pressure: Müller-Hillis maneuver

3.0   Procedure:

   3.1   Instrument(s) used:
      3.1.1   forceps
      3.1.2   vacuum extractor
      3.1.3   Murless or other vectus blade

   3.2   Analgesia/anesthesia

   3.3   Application/checks

   3.4   Traction:
      3.4.1   number of efforts, cup displacement
      3.4.2   manually assisted rotation or spontaneous
      3.4.3   difficulty of extraction
      3.4.4   technique: Saxtorph-Pajot maneuver, etc.
      3.4.5   total period of vacuum application

   3.5   Episiotomy/repair:
      3.5.1   degree of extension, if any
      3.5.2   suture material
      3.5.3   technique of repair

continued

Table II.7   *continued*

4.0   Complications/comments:

    4.1   Apgar scores/neonatal weight

    4.2   Fetal condition:

        4.2.1   resuscitation

        4.2.2   injuries/repair

        4.2.3   cord pH

        4.2.4   other observations

        4.2.5   site of cup application

    4.3   Maternal condition:

        4.3.1   injuries/repair

        4.3.2   estimate blood loss/replacement

        4.3.3   other observations

    4.4   Additional comments (e.g. placenta submitted for examination, etc.)

*These issues are to be considered in all operative vaginal delivery dictations. The comments included are indicated by the circumstances of the individual case

Proper documentation is the best evidence of appropriate professional conduct on behalf of the surgeon in event of subsequent legal investigation of maternal or fetal injury. The bitter experience of many clinicians attests to the fact that accurate and complete documentation at the time of a delivery can eliminate a great deal of difficulty in later recounting or explaining the events surrounding the birth. In such circumstances, a poor record is often a poor defense and it is *always* a professional embarrassment (see Chapter V, Legal issues, Section 4, Documentation).

3.2   Forceps vs. vacuum extraction operations

If presumed fetal jeopardy ('fetal distress') is diagnosed at low station (beyond + 2/5 cm), many traditionally trained practitioners prefer to apply forceps rather than the vacuum extractor. In reviews of published prospective trials, however, there was no demonstrable difference in either safety or speed when either forceps or the vacuum extractor was applied in such situations[3–5,49,50]. Thus, either instrument is appropriate in this setting.

The rules for conduct of an instrumental trial in difficult circumstances are simple. When an emergent delivery is required, and a vaginal operative delivery is elected, the surgeon chooses the most familiar and immediately available instrument[17,28,50-54]. Theoretical concerns aside, under emergent circumstances, greater success and less danger result when instruments are chosen based on operator experience and proven skill. However, it is well to recall that safety and not simply speed is the surgeon's ultimate goal. A methodical approach and *sangfroid* best characterize the obstetric surgeon.

When it is not an emergency, other issues deserve consideration. In outlet operations, assuming adequate analgesia, the vacuum extractor and the forceps are essentially equivalent instruments[6,55,56]. A pudendal block can be administered if forceps are chosen; this can often be omitted for a simple outlet vacuum extraction. As always, it is prudent to reinforce any local anesthesia by vocal reassurance, regardless of the instrument chosen. For outlet procedures one of the polyethylene or silastic/ polyethylene vacuum extractors is the instrument of choice. A rigid metal cup can also be applied as an outlet instrument, but at the risk of producing a chignon.

The most important advantages of vacuum extraction over forceps are in low pelvic procedures involving cranial rotation or mid-pelvic operations when fetal jeopardy is not at issue[50,57,58]. Although true mid-pelvic vaginal forceps operations are now uncommon in general practice, as many newly trained obstetricians have little if any experience with such procedures, they need not be abandoned by experienced practitioners[6,43]. Competent obstetric surgeons can perform mid-pelvic forceps rotations safely with a level of success equal to that of skilled accoucheurs employing the vacuum extractor[59]. However, mid-pelvic forceps rotations should *never* be attempted by an inexperienced surgeon, as, even in experienced hands, the likelihood for maternal injury is greater in mid-cavity forceps operations than with properly conducted vacuum extractions[50,58,60,61-63].

Studies comparing forceps and vacuum extraction for similar indications reveal a mixed but generally consistent pattern (see Chapter IV, Complications and birth injuries, Section 1, Risks: an overview). Fetal scalp injuries and mild postnatal jaundice are more frequent following vacuum extraction operations, while maternal perineal injuries are more likely with forceps deliveries[4,6,52,58,64,65]. Long-term abnormalities in maternal rectal sphincter function do occur, and fistula formation accompanies a small but clinically important percentage of perineal injuries following instrumental delivery[66-71]. Transitory neonatal jaundice and retinal hemorrhage are reported more commonly in vacuum extraction-delivered neonates than in those delivered by forceps. However, these complications are of trivial clinical consequence. Nonetheless, it is important to recall that both the vacuum extractor and the forceps are capable of potentially serious fetal/maternal injury. While rare, such events serve as a constant reminder of the seriousness of purpose and careful technique required by the surgeon in undertaking *any* instrumental delivery.

The vacuum extractor has several important advantages over forceps as a delivery instrument. The cup can be applied and traction exerted with minimal maternal analgesia[4,49,72]. This is particularly useful when the mother refuses a major anesthetic, or when a regional anesthetic has either failed or proven only partially successful. As the vacuum extractor is not applied against the vaginal walls, cranial rotation does not bring the cup into contact with maternal tissues. This minimizes the risk of vaginal vault injuries, especially when rotation accompanies delivery[5,17,58,72]. Third- and fourth-degree perineal lacerations and fetal facial (VII) nerve injuries are also less likely with vacuum extraction, at least in comparison to classic forceps operations[52,71,73]. Unexpectedly, vacuum extraction operations are associated with an increased incidence of shoulder dystocia. This may reflect the preferential use of vacuum procedures in cases of suspected fetopelvic disproportion.

We should not make the mistake that ease of application is an important advantage to vacuum extraction. Admittedly, there is some truth to this claim for simple outlet procedures where the probability of success on the perineum is virtually assured and the effort expended by the surgeon is minimal. However, for procedures above the pelvic floor or with malpositions, the vacuum extractor has exacting requirements for proper application and traction which equal those of forceps procedures. There are significant maternal and fetal risks to both procedures. *All vacuum extractions, regardless of apparent ease, are surgical operations and as such deserve precisely the same close attention to detail as any other obstetric operation.* Any delivery can only be assessed as 'easy' in retrospect. It is a capital error to make a prospective assumption of complete normality about any delivery until it is completed.

Not all vacuum cup designs are equally successful. As an example, Chenoy and Johanson[12] report increased Silc™ Cup failures if 'excess' caput is present. However, where outlet operations are concerned, there is minimal difference between available designs. For such simple outlet procedures, with a normal fetal presentation, any of the available soft cups in any cup size is an appropriate choice. A rigid metal cup of the Bird or O'Neil design would be equally successful. Low pelvic or mid-pelvic operations which do not involve significant asynclitism or posterior positioning are equally well managed by any vacuum instrument. For markedly asynclitic heads in transverse arrest, a metal OP cup or the Mityvac 'M'™ Cup are reasonable choices. If extraction from a direct OP is attempted, an OP metal cup such as the Bird or O'Neil design is clearly superior[4]. The Mityvac 'M'™ may also be employed for an extraction attempt from an OP position, although published clinical data concerning the use of this instrument are scanty[74]. If a posterior or transverse fetal head is more than minimally deflexed, neither the Kobayashi nor the usual plastic disposable extractors can be applied correctly and the likelihood of a traction failure is high[4,75]. In this setting either an OP cup or forceps are the best choices to achieve a vaginal delivery.

3.3   Use of force

The use of force in instrumental delivery is a difficult subject. In general, the obstetric surgeon should augment the mother's voluntary and involuntary efforts with only that force which is minimally required to extract the fetus. Any greater force may accelerate the delivery but also increases the risk of fetal and/or maternal injury. The problem is, how much force is enough?

In vacuum extraction operations, safety is best assured by initially screening instrumental candidates closely for clinical signs of disproportion, and by careful intraoperative cup placement. It is also critical to strictly limit the surgeon's efforts in terms of number of traction efforts, cup displacements, and the total period for cup application. A review of vacuum extraction operations reveals that more than 85% of ultimately successful applications occur with four or fewer traction efforts (Table II.6). The most important rule is that *descent of the fetal head should begin with the initial traction effort.* Failure of prompt descent is the cardinal indication for abandoning a procedure, unless there has been technical failure or misapplication[4,6,76].

As previously discussed, under most circumstances of failed vacuum extraction trial (despite correct application and appropriate technique), a subsequent trial of forceps is *not* recommended[6,43,47]. Similarly, a failed forceps trial is a contraindication to a subsequent trial of vacuum extraction.

3.4 Training deficiencies

Training in vacuum extraction for the great majority of US practitioners is incomplete or deficient[77]. This is a particular challenge to medical educators. Minimization of risk in the use of vacuum extraction is dependent upon expert instruction, adequate experience, and strict adherence to protocol[4,6,7,78,79]. It is to be emphasized that correct vacuum technique is not learned from package inserts, video presentations or textbooks alone. Such aids should only serve to parallel and reinforce competent, direct instruction by an experienced practitioner. Surgery is best taught by surgeons, with 'hands-on' instruction followed by extensive practice. Textbooks provide background information, and suggest new approaches, or review the clinical experiences of others but cannot instruct in judgment, forbearance, or the judicious use of force.

Nonetheless, when formal training programs are not available, self-education must suffice, combining clinical and textbook instruction. The best rule is to commence with simple outlet extractions involving neither cranial malpositioning nor presumed fetal jeopardy/distress. Thereafter, progressive graduation to more complex procedures is possible, once confidence and facility with easier operations have been achieved. Difficult vacuum procedures should *never* be attempted without a background of exact instruction, regardless of the surgeon's prior experience with forceps operations. Accoucheurs should not expect that skill in forceps operations will automatically be translated into prompt success with the vacuum extractor.

3.5 Effects of anesthesia

In most American obstetrical services, epidural blockade is the anesthetic of choice for pain relief during labor. Despite controversy, it is generally accepted that epidural anesthesia, as currently practiced, increases the likelihood of instrumental delivery and Cesarean delivery[20,25,80–89].

Some facts are generally conceded. Epidurals have physiological effects that potentially alter the course of labor. Epidural-induced vasodilation can lead to maternal hypotension. The usual brachial artery blood pressure determinations do not necessarily reflect the extent of this uterine hypoperfusion. Adverse fetal consequences are reduced by continuous attention to adequate maternal hydration and lateral recumbency positioning[80]. However, adequate maternal pain relief also enhances co-operation, lessens maternal exhaustion, and reduces the stress-related elevations in catecholamines that accompany labor[90]. Adverse effects of epidurally administered pain relief agents on the neonate are minimal.

Epidurals transiently reduce spontaneous uterine contraction force and in most, but not all studies, prolong the first stage of labor slightly, even when oxytocin is administered. However, this effect is generally of minor consequence unless the epidural is administered prior to the active phase of labor. The potential effect(s) of epidural anesthesia on labor progress remain controversial and no clear consensus of opinion exists[87–89,91,92].

The major adverse effects of epidural blockade arise during the second stage of labor. Poor second-stage progress under epidural blockade occurs because the block interferes with voluntary and involuntary maternal expulsive efforts by changing muscle tone and attenuating reflex arcs[83,87,89]. Normally, uterine contractions increase in strength with cranial descent as the second stage progresses. Especially marked in unmedicated labors, those more intense uterine contractions occur at or near full dilation, and are usually followed rapidly by the mother's spontaneous urge to bear down (transition phase). This effect is believed to result from stimulation of sensory output by the pelvic autonomic nerves and the endogenous release of oxytocin[91,93]. Epidural anesthesia interferes with this process by blockade of nerve transmission. The more profound the motor and sensory blockade, the greater is the likelihood of inhibiting this bearing-down reflex[94,95]. If dense epidural anesthesia is administered, the clinical result is prolongation of the second stage, interference with cranial descent/rotation, and an increased likelihood of instrumental delivery[86].

It is not clear that consistently effective analgesia can be provided throughout the second stage of labor without *some* increase in the incidence of instrumental and/or Cesarean delivery[83,84,87–89,95–97]. The question is one of degree. There is the strong suggestion that different management protocols for oxytocin and epidural use make it possible to provide adequate analgesia for most labors *and* permit near normal labor progress[86,88,95,96,98]. Oxytocin augmentation should be used without hesitation in the second stage if progress under epidural blockade is slow and disproportion is excluded by clinical examination[96].

Accumulated clinical experience suggests that anesthetic techniques administering a combination of opioids and local anesthetics and other agents by continuous peridural infusion provide adequate pain relief for

41

both vaginal delivery and vaginal instrumentation, with minimal affect on second-stage labor[85,88,99,100]. There is active clinical experimentation in this field and the development of new epidural protocols providing labor analgesia while avoiding major motor blockade can be confidently predicted.

Coaching, administration of oxytocin, and extension of the time allowed for second stage when using epidural anesthesia are helpful in promoting either spontaneous delivery or in achieving a lower station of the fetal head prior to an instrumental delivery[6,24,101–103]. Voluntary bearing down in the second stage is best deferred until spontaneous descent occurs or until the mother perceives pelvic pressure and the spontaneous desire to push[104]. This more closely simulates normal second-stage progression. Prolonged maternal expulsive efforts, arbitrarily beginning at full dilation, despite being widely practiced, are often of limited benefit in speeding descent. Delayed pushing, squatting, or partial upright positioning may be beneficial in gaining station. Such practices avoid prolonged and exhaustive maternal expulsive efforts[102,105,106].

With these changes in both obstetric and anesthesia management, it is possible to convert many mid-pelvic procedures into simple low pelvic or outlet operations[95]. The aim for both the obstetrician and the anesthesiologist must be to provide analgesia for labor and delivery, not surgical anesthesia. A surgical level of anesthesia for labor is unnecessary and inhibits effective labor progress. As Bailey and co-workers have shown[107,108], when appropriate alterations in both obstetric and anesthesia management are made, use of epidural anesthesia need not be associated with major changes in the rate of either assisted or Cesarean delivery (Figure II.7).

3.6 Clinical evaluation of pelvic adequacy

Evaluation of progress in labor, the appropriateness of operative intervention, as well as the correct application of any instrument, depend on a correct diagnosis of the station, attitude, and position of the fetal head. The central clinical problem is that of dystocia.

A number of terms are used to describe labor dystocia. The most common are cephalopelvic disproportion (CPD) and failure to progress (FTP)[109]. Dystocia results either from true or relative disparity between the maternal bony pelvis and the fetal head, or a combination of these

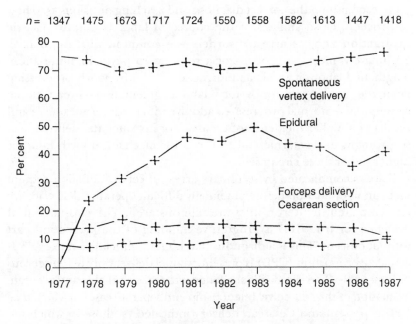

Figure II.7 Effects of the introduction of an epidural service at the Dorcaster Royal Infirmary, 1977–1987, by mode of delivery. From reference 107 with permission

conditions[25]. In most instances the problem is failure to progress, or 'relative CPD'. This arises from inadequate uterine powers, ineffectual maternal bearing-down efforts, or a complex of fetal malpositioning, maternal soft tissue and cervical resistance combined with other problems[25,110,111]. In current practice, a true contracted pelvis with an average-sized fetus is a rare cause of dystocia. The more common problem is a macrosomic fetus in an average-sized pelvis or the malpositioning of an average-sized fetus in an otherwise adequate pelvis[110–113]. As ordinarily practiced, clinical pelvimetry is of limited help and usually unnecessary in deciding which patients should have either a trial of labor or receive oxytocin stimulation, except in extreme cases. Anatomical disproportion is uncommon and surprisingly difficult to diagnose. Contracted pelves are rare in modern practice unless there is a maternal anomaly (e.g. achondroplasia) or a history of prior pelvic fracture. However, if progress under adequate oxytocin stimulation is tardy or if a trial of instrumental delivery is contemplated, a *comprehensive* evaluation of pelvic adequacy is required, as discussed below[7,102,114,115].

43

In establishing the correct diagnosis and reaching decisions as to how to proceed, close analysis of the course of labor is helpful. Classic protraction and/or arrest disorders are common with dystocia[116]. Fortunately, most cases of dystocia respond to oxytocin stimulation, lengthened labor or simple amniorrhexis[109,117–119]. In poorly progressing labor, the requirement for oxytocin labor augmentation – even with the resumption of normal progress – is additive with epidural anesthesia and results in a higher incidence of Cesarean or instrumental delivery. Not surprisingly, the maternal and fetal risk for mechanical birth injury is higher under these circumstances.

Labors complicated by secondary arrest of cervical dilation require meticulous evaluation before potentially difficult operative deliveries are contemplated or uterotronics are administered. The classic clinical evidence for true CPD is progressive molding of the presenting part without descent. This is a diagnosis that is often difficult to make[43,120]. If actual disproportion (CPD) is present, vaginal delivery proves dangerous or impossible. The clinician's challenge is to make a reliable and accurate evaluation of this fetopelvic relationship and separate cases in which true CPD is present and Cesarean delivery indicated vs. those in which the dystocia is *relative* and uterine stimulation or operative vaginal delivery are appropriate procedures.

If heavy cranial molding is present, the clinician has difficulty in determining whether the mass of the head is descending or if simply molding and edema account for the movement of the presenting part deeper into the maternal pelvis. In this setting, station cannot be accurately judged based solely on palpation of the leading edge of the presenting part and other clinical findings become more important[6,7,44,79,121,122].

Initially, it is prudent to perform Leopold's maneuvers abdominally and follow with the Müller–Hillis maneuver (MHM) during a careful pelvic examination[123]. This assists the clinician in judging the degree of cranial molding and fetopelvic capacity. If on vaginal bimanual examination the presenting part fails to descend with fundal pressure (MHM) and marked cranial molding is present (Philpott–Vacca maneuver described subsequently)[4,5], pelvic adequacy is suspect. In this circumstance, instrumental delivery should proceed with great circumspection or, best, be abandoned altogether. Similarly, abdominal palpation may discover additional contraindications to instrumentation: a high presenting part, a face or brow presentation, or a fetal head overriding the pubic symphysis.

Other clinical findings are also helpful[121,124]. Failure of the fetal head to fill the posterior hollow of the sacrum is a strong suggestion that the head lies higher than expected and has not negotiated the midpelvis. Similarly, failure to palpate the fetal ear easily also suggests high station. Careful estimation of the extent of the fetal head situated abdominally is also useful. In this technique, the extent of cranial descent into the pelvis is estimated in fifths. Engagement of the fetal head has occurred when no more than one-fifth of the fetal head remains palpable abdominally. Obviously, anesthesia, patient size, and her compliance contribute to the success of such examinations.

Philpott[113] and Vacca[4,5] describe an additional and useful technique of gauging the extent of disproportion. In this method, the degree of cranial molding is estimated by judging the overlap of the fetal cranial bones at the occipito–parietal and parietal–parietal junctions (Figure II.8). The extent of this overlap and the ease of reduction by simple digital pressure are noted. If the bones are overlapping and cannot be reduced easily by simple digital pressure, molding is judged as advanced or extreme or and disproportion is likely to be present. Instrumental deliveries are likely to fail or prove dangerous under such circumstances and are usually best avoided or, if attempted, reserved for a wary approach by only the most experienced.

Radiographic pelvimetry was once popular in evaluating cephalic presentations. However, as currently practiced, classic X-ray pelvimetry has little, if any, role, to play in evaluating labor progress or suspected disproportion[25,125]. The positive predictive value of the measurements are simply unacceptably poor and do not serve as a valid guide for clinical management of accoucheurs.

Unfortunately and somewhat unexpectedly, neither ultrasonic estimations of fetal weight nor calculation of ratios between specific fetal measurements have proven useful in judging the risk of traumatic delivery. This is largely due to the relative inaccuracy of these methods in estimating the size of infants and relating these measurements to pelvic capacity (see Chapter IV, Complications and birth injuries, Section 2.5, Shoulder dystocia and Chapter VI, Risk assessment, Section 2.4, Fetal macrosomia). Nonetheless, bedside real-time ultrasonic examinations are useful in evaluating fetal presentation and, to some extent, station. The plane of the fetal orbits is normally identified with ease, especially when the station is high and the position is occiput posterior[126]. Real-time ultrasound is also helpful in the version and extraction of the second infant in twin deliveries.

45

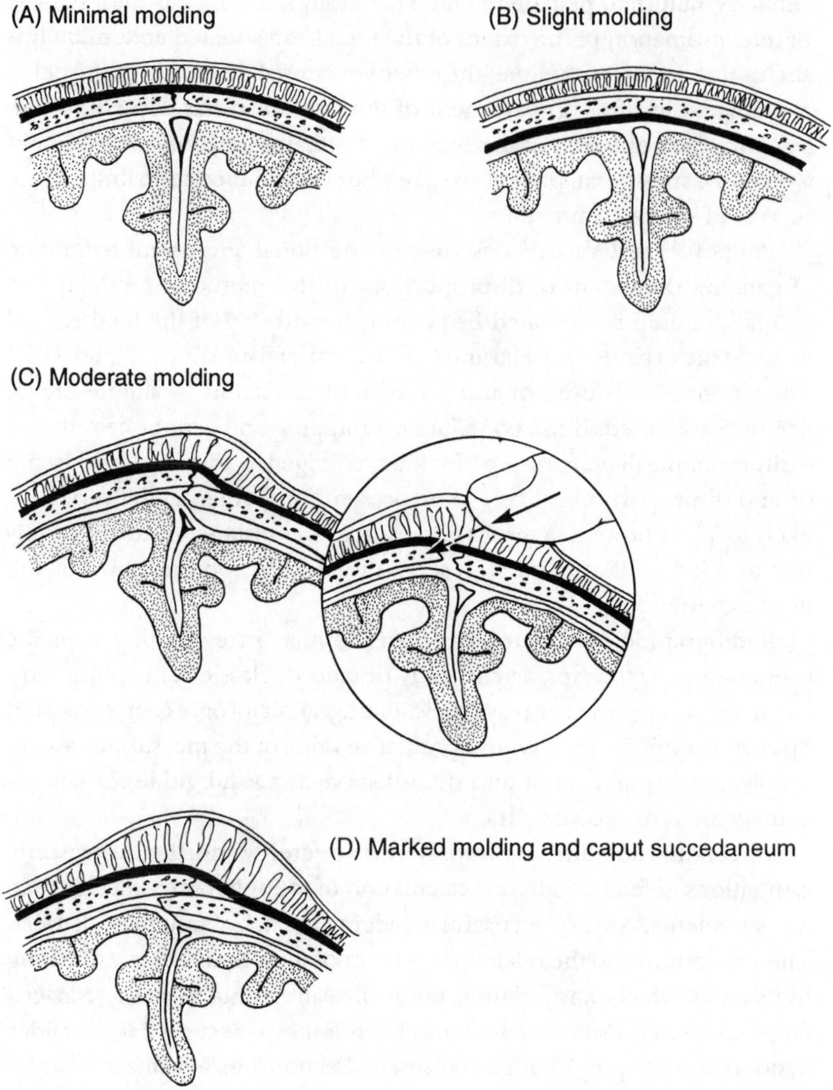

Figure II.8 Clinical evaluation of cranial molding by digital examination. As molding progresses from minimal (A) through slight (B) to moderate (C) and finally to marked (D) the cranial bones progressively overlap and additional caput succedaneum is formed. Illustration (C) indicates how digital palpation judges the extent of cranial bone overlap and its reduction. (Redrawn from Vacca[4])

Provided absolute disproportion and malpresentation have been excluded in cephalic presentations, and progress is poor, the best measure of pelvic adequacy is a trial of oxytocin labor stimulation under close maternal/fetal observation[7,115,127]. Oxytocin can safely be administered to nulliparas by various standard protocols. Dystocia in multiparous patients requires special care, as their risks of oxytocin stimulation are greater.

Trials of labor under oxytocin augmentation require close attention to possible maternal and fetal distress[118]. In cases of dystocia, in common American practice, the adequacy of uterine activity is documented by continuous monitoring using a pressure catheter or transducer[25,98,128]. However, such invasive monitoring may not be required in all cases. The Dublin group has safely used oxytocin stimulation in thousands of cases with 'one-on-one' nursing/midwifery clinical observation without use of electronic detectors for uterine activity[127]. In any event, close clinical observation is essential. Labor progress is judged by serial vaginal examinations with careful recording of cervical dilation, station, and position of the fetal head. Close surveillance is prudent in pregnancies complicated by arrest disorders but the risks of labor stimulation should not be over-emphasized. In such cases, Bottoms[117] observed neither a higher incidence of depressed infants (based on Apgar scores) nor an increase in perinatal mortality, as determined by electronic monitoring.

If advancement of the fetal head ceases following adequate oxytocin stimulation, maternal encouragement, and/or positioning, the clinician must decide between modes of operative delivery – either Cesarean delivery or a trial of instrumental delivery. In this setting, prolonging labor is not an option – a definitive surgical intervention is required to achieve delivery.

Knowledge of pelvic architecture and an appreciation of the total clinical setting assist in deciding if either instrumental or Cesarean delivery is best and which procedure(s) are technically possible. For example, a molded but deflexed occiput posterior head of a suspected macrosomic baby at + 2/5 cm station in a woman with a gynecoid pelvis may lead to vacuum extraction failure. Here, consideration of Cesarean delivery or possibly a forceps trial is appropriate. Alternatively, a fetus presenting as an occiput anterior, in a well-flexed position at + 3/5 cm station in a nullipara with no anesthesia is a good candidate for vacuum extraction. As always, the reasons for whatever choice is made must be carefully recorded in the medical record (see Chapter V, Legal issues, Section 4, Documentation).

REFERENCES

1. Radcliffe, W. (1989). *Milestones in Midwifery and The Secret Instrument*, p. 55. (San Francisco: Norman Publishing)
2. Dewees, W.P. (1826). *A Compendius System of Midwifery, Chiefly Designed to Facilitate the Inquiries of Those Who May be Pursuing this Branch of Study*, p. xii. (Philadelphia: H.C. Carey & I. Lea)
3. Vacca, A. and Keirse, M.J.N.C. (1989). Instrumental vaginal delivery. In Chalmers, I., Eukin, M. and Keirse, M.J.N.C. (eds.) *Effective Care in Pregnancy and Childbirth*, pp. 1216–33. (Oxford: Oxford University Press)
4. Vacca, A. (1992). *Handbook of Vacuum Extraction in Obstetric Practice*. (London: Edward Arnold)
5. Vacca, A. (1990). The place of the vacuum extractor in modern obstetric practice. *Fet. Med. Rev.*, **2**, 103–22
6. O'Grady, J.P. (1988). *Modern Instrumental Delivery*. (Baltimore: Williams & Wilkins)
7. O'Grady, J.P. and Gimovsky, M.L. (1993). Instrumental delivery: a lost art? In Studd, J. (ed.) *Progress in Obstetrics and Gynaecology*, vol. 10, pp. 183–212. (New York: Churchill-Livingstone)
8. Bird, G.C. (1969). Modification of Malmström's vacuum extractor. *Br. Med. J.*, **3**, 526
9. O'Neil, A.G.B., Skull, E. and Michael, C. (1981). A new method of traction for the vacuum cup. *Aust. NZ. J. Obstet. Gynaecol.*, **21**, 24–5
10. Hofmeyr, G.J., Gobetz, L., Sonnendecker, E.W. and Turner, M.J. (1990). New design rigid and soft vacuum extractor cups: a preliminary comparison of traction forces. *Br. J. Obstet. Gynaecol.*, **97**, 681–5
11. Laufe, L.E. and Berkus, M.D. (1992). *Assisted Vaginal Delivery*. (New York: McGraw-Hill, Inc.)
12. Chenoy, R. and Johanson, R. (1992). A randomized prospective study comparing delivery with metal and silicone rubber vacuum extractor cups. *Br. J. Obstet. Gynaecol.*, **99**, 360–3
13. Kuit, J.A., Eppinga, N.G., Wallenburg, N.C. and Huiskeshoven, F.J. (1993). A randomized comparison of vacuum extraction delivery with a rigid and a pliable cup. *Obstet. Gynecol.*, **82**, 280–4
14. Cohn, M., Barclay, C., Fraser, R., Zaklama, M., Johanson, R., Anderson, D. and Walker, C. (1989). A multicentre randomized trial comparing delivery with a silicone rubber cup and rigid metal vacuum extractor cups. *Br. J. Obstet. Gynaecol.*, **96**, 545–51
15. Hammarström, M., Csemiczky, G. and Belfrage, P. (1986). Comparison between the conventional Malmström extractor and a new extractor with silastic cup. *Acta Obstet. Gynecol. Scand.*, **65**, 791–2
16. Loghis, C., Pyrgiotis, E., Panayotopoulos, N., Batalias, L., Salamelekis, E. and Zourlas, P.A. (1992). Comparison between metal cup and silicone rubber cup vacuum extractor. *Eur. J. Obstet. Gynecol. Reprod. Biol.*, **45**, 173–6

17. Johanson, R., Pusey, J., Livera, N. and Jones, P. (1989). North Staffordshire/ Wigan assisted delivery trial. *Br. J. Obstet. Gynaecol.*, **96**, 537–44

18. Hastie, S.J. and MacLean, A.B. (1986). Comparison of the use of the Silastic obstetric vacuum extractor to Kielland's forceps. *Asia Oceania J. Obstet. Gynecol.*, **12**, 63–8

19. Meyer, L., Mailloux, J., Marcoux, S., Blanchet, P. and Meyer, F. (1987). Maternal and neonatal morbidity in instrumental deliveries with the Kobayashi vacuum extractor and low forceps. *Acta Obstet. Gynecol. Scand.*, **66**, 643–7

20. American College of Obstetricians and Gynecologists (1994). *Operative Vaginal Delivery*. Technical Bulletin No. 196. (Washington DC: American College of Obstetricians and Gynecologists)

21. American College of Obstetricians and Gynecologists (1991). *Operative Vaginal Delivery*. Technical Bulletin No. 152. (Washington DC: American College of Obstetricians and Gynecologists)

22. American College of Obstetricians and Gynecologists Committee on Obstetrics (1989). *Maternal and Fetal Medicine: Obstetric Forceps*. Committee Opinion No. 71. (Washington DC: American College of Obstetricians and Gynecologists)

23. Hagadorn-Freathy, A.S., Yeomans, E.R. and Hankins, G.D. (1991). Validation of the 1988 ACOG forceps classification system. *Obstet. Gynecol.*, **77**, 356–60

24. Derham, R.J., Crowhurst, J. and Crowther, C. (1991). The second stage of labour: durational dilemmas. *Aust. NZ J. Obstet. Gynaecol.*, **31**, 31–6

25. American College of Obstetricians and Gynecologists (1989). *Dystocia*. Technical Bulletin No. 137. (Washington DC: American College of Obstetricians and Gynecologists)

26. DeLee, J.B. (1920). The prophylactic forceps operation. *Am. J. Obstet. Gynecol.*, **1**, 34–44.

27. Niswander, K.R. and Gordond, M. (1973). Safety of the low-forceps operations. *Am. J. Obstet. Gynecol.*, **117**, 619–30

28. Yancey, M.K., Herpolsheimer, A., Jordan, G.D., Benson, W.L. and Brady, K. (1991). Maternal and neonatal effects of outlet forceps delivery compared with spontaneous vaginal delivery in term pregnancies. *Obstet. Gynecol.*, **78**, 646–50

29. Bishop, E.H., Israel, S.L. and Briscoe, L.C. (1965). Obstetric influences on the premature infant's first year of development. *Obstet. Gynecol.*, **26**, 628–35

30. Schwartz, D.B., Miodovnik, M. and Lavin, J.P. (1983). Neonatal outcome among low birth weight infants delivered spontaneously or by low forceps. *Obstet. Gynecol.*, **62**, 283–6

31. Nyirjesy, I. and Pierce, W.E. (1964). Perinatal mortality and maternal morbidity in spontaneous and forceps vaginal deliveries. *Am. J. Obstet. Gynecol.*, **89**, 568–78

32. Schindler, N.R. (1991). Importance of the placenta and cord in the defense of neurologically impaired infant claims. *Arch. Pathol. Lab. Med.*, 115, 685–7

33. Gilstrap, L.C. 3rd, Leveno, K.J., Burns, J., Williams, M.L. and Little, B.B. (1989). Diagnosis of birth asphyxia on the basis of fetal pH, Apgar score, and minimal cerebral dysfunction. *Am. J. Obstet. Gynecol.*, 161, 825–30

34. Humphrey, M.D., Chang, A., Wood, E.C., Morgan, S. and Hounslow, D. (1974). A decrease in fetal pH during the second stage of labour, when conducted in the dorsal position. *J. Obstet. Gynaecol. Br. Commonw.*, 81, 600–2

35. Rosemann, G.W.E. (1969). Vacuum extraction of premature infants. *S. Afr. J. Obstet. Gynaecol.*, 7, 10–12

36. Sanchez-Ramos, L., Morales, R. and Cullen, M.T. (1992). Vacuum extraction in preterm infants: a case control study. In *Proceedings of Annual Meeting of Society of Perinatal Obstetricians*, Abstr. No. 450, p. 332

37. Roberts, I.F. and Stone, M. (1978). Fetal hemorrhage: complication of vacuum extractor after fetal blood sampling. *Am. J. Obstet. Gynecol.*, 132, 109.

38. Thiery, M. (1979). Letter to the Editor. Fetal hemorrhage following blood sampling and use of vacuum extraction. *Am. J. Obstet. Gynecol.*, 134, 231

39. Solomons, E. (1962). Delivery of the head with the Malmström vacuum extractor during cesarean section. *Obstet. Gynecol.*, 19, 201–3

40. Bercovici, B. (1980). Use of the vacuum extractor for head delivery at cesarean section. *Isr. J. Med. Sci.*, 16, 201–3

41. Pelosi, M.A. and Apuzzio, J. (1984). Use of the soft, silicone obstetric vacuum cups for the delivery of the fetal head at cesarean section. *J. Reprod. Med.*, 29, 289–92

42. Lowe, B. (1987). Fear of failure: a place for the trial of instrumental delivery. *Br. J. Obstet. Gynaecol.*, 94, 60–6

43. de Villiers, V.P. (1991). Obstetric forceps after a failed ventouse application. *S. Afr. Med. J.*, 80, 301

44. Saropala, N. and Chaturachinda, K. (1991). Failed instrumental delivery; Ramathibodi Hospital 1980–1988. *Int. J. Gynecol. Obstet.*, 36, 203–7

45. Pusey, J. and Hodge, C. (1991). Maternal impressions of forceps or the Silc-cup. *Br. J. Obstet. Gynaecol.*, 98, 487–8

46. Sjostedt, J.E. (1967). The vacuum extractor and forceps in obstetrics: a clinical study. *Acta Obstet. Gynecol. Scand.*, 46, 203–8

47. Pelosi, M.A. and Pelosi, M.A. III (1992). Letter to the Editor. A randomized comparison of assisted vaginal delivery by obstetric forceps and polyethylene vacuum cup. *Obstet. Gynecol.*, 79, 638–9

48. Cyr, R.M., Usher, R.H. and McLean, C.M. (1984). Changing patterns of birth asphyxia and trauma over 20 years. *Am. J. Obstet. Gynecol.*, 148, 490–8

49. Vacca, A., Grant, A., Wyatt, G. and Chalmers, I. (1983). Portsmouth operative delivery trial: a comparison of vacuum extraction and forceps delivery. *Br. J. Obstet. Gynaecol.*, 90, 1107–12

50. Chalmers, J.A. and Chalmers, I. (1989). The obstetric vacuum extractor is the instrument of first choice for operative vaginal delivery. *Br. J. Obstet. Gynaecol.*, **96**, 505–6

51. Pearse, W.H. (1965). Forceps versus spontaneous vaginal delivery. *Clin. Obstet. Gynecol.*, **8**, 813–21

52. Punnonen, R., Avo, P., Kuukankorpi, A. and Pystynen, P. (1986). Fetal and maternal effects of forceps and vacuum extraction. *Br. J. Obstet. Gynaecol.*, **93**, 1132–5

53. Vacca, A. and Kierse, M.J.N.C. In Chalmers, I., Enkin, M. and Keirse, M.J.N.C. (eds.) pp. 1216–34. Instrumental vaginal delivery. In *Effective Care in Pregnancy and Childbirth*. (Oxford: Oxford University Press)

54. Lasbrey, A.H., Orchard, C.D. and Critchon, D. (1964). A study of the relative merits and scope for vacuum extraction as opposed to forceps delivery. *S. Afr. J. Obstet. Gynecol.*, **2**, 1–3

55. Fall, O., Ryden, G., Finnström, K. and Finnström, O. (1986). Forceps or vacuum extraction? A comparison of effects on the newborn infant. *Acta Obstet. Gynecol. Scand.*, **65**, 75–80

56. Livnat, E.J., Fejgin, M., Scommegna, A., Bieniarz, J. and Burd, L. (1978). Neonatal acid-base balance in spontaneous and instrumental vaginal deliveries. *Obstet. Gynecol.*, **52**, 549–51

57. De Jonge, E.T.M. and Lindeque, B.G. (1991). A properly conducted trial of a ventouse can prevent unexpected failure of instrumental delivery. *S. Afr. Med. J.*, **79**, 545–6

58. Broekhuizen, F.F., Washington, J.M., Johnson, F. and Hamilton, P.R. (1987). Vacuum extraction versus forceps delivery: indications and complications, 1979–1984. *Obstet. Gynecol.*, **69**, 338–42

59. Herabutya, Y., O-Prasertsawat, P. and Boonrangsimant, P. (1988). Kielland's forceps or ventouse – a comparison. *Br. J. Obstet. Gynaecol.*, **95**, 483–7

60. Robertson, P.A., Laros, R.K. and Zhao, R.L. (1990). Neonatal and maternal outcome in low-pelvic and midpelvic operative deliveries. *Am. J. Obstet. Gynecol.*, **162**, 1436–42

61. Bashore, R.A., Phillips, W.H. Jr and Brinkman, C.R. (1990). A comparison of the morbidity of midforceps and cesarean delivery. *Am. J. Obstet. Gynecol.*, **162**, 1428–35

62. Cibilis, L.A. and Ringler, G.E. (1990). Evaluation of midforceps delivery as an alternative. *J. Perinat. Med.*, **18**, 5–11

63. Baerthlein, W.C., Moodley, S. and Stinson, S.K. (1986). Comparison of maternal and neonatal morbidity in midforceps delivery and midpelvic vacuum extraction. *Obstet. Gynecol.*, **67**, 594–7

64. Johanson, R.B., Rice, C., Doyle, M., Arthur, J., Anyanwu, L., Ibrahim, J., Warwick, A., Ridman, C.W. and O'Brien . P.M. (1993). A randomised prospective study comparing the new vacuum extractor policy with forceps delivery. *Br. J. Obstet. Gynaecol.*, **100**, 524–30

65. Greis, J.B., Bieniarz, J. and Scommegna, A. (1981). Comparison of maternal and fetal effects of vacuum extraction with forceps or cesarean deliveries. *Obstet. Gynecol.*, **57**, 571–7

66. Gass, M.S., Dunn, C. and Stys, S.J. (1986). Effect of episiotomy on the frequency of vaginal outlet lacerations. *J. Reprod. Med.*, **31**, 240–4

67. Thorp, J.M. Jr, Bowers, W.A. Jr, Brame, R.G. and Cefab, R. (1987). Selected use of mid-line episiotomy: effect on perineal trauma. *Obstet. Gynecol.*, **70**, 260–2

68. Haadem, K., Dahlstrom, J.A., Ling, L. and Ohrlander, S. (1987). Anal sphincter function after delivery rupture. *Obstet. Gynecol.*, **70**, 53–6

69. Sultan, A.H., Kamm, M.A., Bartram, C.I. *et al.* (1993). Anal sphincter trauma during instrumental delivery. *Int. J. Gynecol. Obstet.*, **43**, 263–70

70. Combs, C.A., Robertson, P.A. and Laros, R.K., Jr. (1990). Risk factors for third-degree perineal lacerations in forceps and vacuum deliveries. *Am. J. Obstet. Gynecol.*, **163**, 100–4

71. Sultan, A.H., Kamm, M.A., Hudson, C.N. and Bartram, C.I. (1994). Third degree tears: incidence, risk factors, and poor clinical outcome after primary sphincter repair. *Br. Med. J.*, **308**, 887–91

72. Bird, G.C. (1982). The use of the vacuum extractor. *Clin. Obstet. Gynaecol.*, **9**, 641–61

73. William, M.C., Knuppel, R.A., O'Brien, W.F., Weiss, A. and Kanarek, K.S. (1991). A randomized comparison of assisted vaginal delivery by obstetric forceps and polyethylene vacuum cup. *Obstet. Gynecol.*, **78**, 789–94

74. Ross, M.G. (1994). Vacuum delivery by soft cup extraction. *Contemp. Ob/Gyn.*, **39**, 48–53

75. Vacca, A. (1993). Letter to the Editor. Effect of angular traction on the performance of modern vacuum extractors. *Am. J. Obstet. Gynecol.*, **169**, 748–9

76. Bird, G.C. (1976). The importance of flexion in vacuum extractor delivery. *Br. J. Obstet. Gynaecol.*, **83**, 194–200

77. Iffy, L., Lancet, M. and Kessler, I. (1984). The vacuum extractor. In Iffy, L. and Charles, D. (eds.) *Operative Perinatology: Invasive Obstetric Techniques*, pp. 582–93. (New York: Macmillan Publishing)

78. Plauche, W.C. (1979). Fetal cranial injuries related to delivery with the Malmström vacuum extractor. *Obstet. Gynecol.*, **53**, 750–7

79. Nargolkar, S.M., O'Grady, J.P. and Gimovsky, M.L. (1993). Modern vaginal instrumental delivery. In Krishna, U. and Daftary, S. (eds.) *Pregnancy at Risk: Current Concepts*, pp. 427–35. (Bombay: The Federation of Obstetric and Gynecological Societies of India)

80. Reynolds, F. (1989). Epidural analgesia in obstetrics: pros and cons for mother and baby. *Br. Med. J.*, **299**, 751–2

81. Reynolds, F. (1991). Pain relief in labour. In Studd, J. (ed.) *Progress in Obstetrics*

and Gynaecology, vol. 9, pp. 131–48. (Edinburgh: Churchill-Livingstone)

82. Kaminski, H.M., Stafl, A. and Aiman, J. (1987). The effect of analgesia on the frequency of instrumental obstetric delivery. *Obstet. Gynecol.*, **69**, 770–3

83. Thorp, J.A., Parisi, J.M., Boylan, P.C. and Johnston, D.A. (1989). The effect of continuous epidural analgesia on cesarean section for dystocia in nulliparous women. *Am. J. Obstet. Gynecol.*, **161**, 670–5

84. Garbaciak, J.A. (1990). Labor and delivery: anesthesia, induction of labor, malpresentation, and operative delivery. *Curr. Opin. Obstet. Gynecol.*, **2**, 773–9

85. Chestnut, D.H. (1991). Epidural anesthesia and instrumental vaginal delivery. *J. Anesthesiol.*, **74**, 805–8

86. O'Grady, J.P. and Youngstrom, P. (1990). Must epidurals always imply instrumental delivery? *Contemp. Ob/Gyn.*, **35**, 19–27

87. Thorp, J.A., Eckert, L.O., Ang, M.S., Johnston, D.A., Peaceman, A.M. and Parisi, V.M. (1991). Epidural analgesia and cesarean section for dystocia: risk factors in nulliparas. *Am. J. Perinatol.*, **8**, 402–10

88. Chestnut, D.H., Vincent, R.D., McGrath, J.M., Vincent, R.D. Jr., Penning, D.H., Choi, W.W., Bates, J.N. and McFarlane, C. (1994). Does early administration of epidural analgesia affect obstetric outcome in nulliparous women who are receiving intravenous oxytocin? *Anesthesiology*, **80**, 1193–200

89. Thorp, J.A., Hu, D.H., Albin, R.M. *et al.* (1993). The effect of intrapartum epidural analgesia in nulliparous labor: a randomized, controlled, prospective trial. *Am. J. Obstet. Gynecol.*, **169**, 851–8

90. Shnider, S.M., Abboud, T.K., Artal, R., Henriksen, E.H., Stefani, S.J. and Levinson, G. (1972). Maternal catecholamines decrease during labor after lumbar anesthesia. *Am. J. Obstet. Gynecol.*, **147**, 166–75

91. Bates, R.G., Helm, C.W., Duncan, A. and Edmonds, D.K. (1985). Uterine activity in the second stage of labour and the effect of epidural anesthesia. *Br. J. Obstet. Gynaecol.*, **92**, 1246–50

92. Johnson, W.L., Winter, W.W., Eng, M., Bonica, J.J. and Hunter, C.A. (1972). Effect of pudendal, spinal, and peridural block anesthesia on the second stage of labor. *Am. J. Obstet. Gynecol.*, **113**, 166–75

93. Goodfellow, C.R., Hull, M.G.R., Swaab, D., Dogsteron, J.J. and Burgis, R.M. (1983) Oxytocin deficiency at delivery with epidural analgesia. *Br. J. Obstet. Gynaecol.*, **90**, 214–19

94. Thornburn, J. and Moir, D.D. (1981). Extradural analgesia: the influence of volume and concentration of bupivicaine on the mode of delivery, analgesia efficacy and motor block. *Br. J. Anaesthesiol.*, **53**, 933–9

95. Doughty, A. (1969). Selective epidural analgesia and the forceps rate. *Br. J. Anaesthesiol.*, **41**, 1058–62

96. Saunders, N.J., Spiby, H., Gilbert, L., Fraser, R.B., Hall, J.M., Mutton, P.M., Jackson, A. and Edmonds, D.K. (1989). Oxytocin infusion during second stage of labour in primiparous women using epidural analgesia: a randomised double blind placebo controlled study. *Br. Med. J.*, **299**, 1423–6

97. Phillips, K.C. and Thomas, T.A. (1983). Second stage of labour with or without extradural analgesia. *Anaesthesia*, **38**, 972–6

98. Neuhoff, D., Burks, S. and Porreco, R.P. (1989). Cesarean birth for failed progress in labor. *Obstet. Gynecol.*, **73**, 915–20

99. Youngstrom, P., Sedensky, M. and Frankmann, D. (1988). Continuous epidural infusion of low-dose bupivicaine-fentanyl for labor analgesia. *Anesthesiology*, **69**, A686

100. Vertommen, J.D., Vandermeulen, E., Van Aken, H., Vaes, L., Soelens, M., Van Steenberge, A., Mourisse, P., Willaert, J., Noorduin, H. and Devlieger, H. (1991). The effects of the addition of sufentanil ot 0.125% bupivicaine on the quality of analgesia during labor and on the incidence of instrumental deliveries. *J. Anesthesiol.*, **74**, 805–8

101. Drife, J.O. (1983). Kielland or Caesar? *Br. Med. J.*, **287**, 309–10

102. Crawford, J.S. (1983). The stages and phases of labour: an outworn nomenclature that invites hazard. *Lancet*, **ii**, 271–2

103. Cohen, W.R. (1983). The pelvic division of labor. In Cohen, W.R. and Friedman, E.A. (eds.) *Management of Labor*, pp. 41–64. (Baltimore: University Park Press)

104. Sleep, J., Robert, J. and Chalmers, I. (1989). Care during the second stage of labour. In Chalmers, I., Eukin, M. and Kierse, M.J.N.C. (eds.) *Effective Care in Pregnancy and Childbirth*, pp. 1129–45. (Oxford: Oxford University Press)

105. Gardosi, J., Hutson, B. and Lynch, C. (1989). Randomized controlled trial of squatting in the second stage of labour. *Lancet*, **ii**, 74–7

106. Maresh, M., Choong, K.H. and Beard, R.W. (1983). Delayed pushing with lumbar epidural analgesia in labour. *Br. J. Obstet. Gynaecol.*, **90**, 623–7

107. Bailey, P.W. and Howard, F.A. (1983). Forum. Epidural analgesia and forceps delivery: laying a bogey. *Anaesthesia*, **38**, 282–5

108. Bailey, P.W. (1989). Epidural anesthesia and instrumental delivery. *Anaesthesia*, **44**, 171–2

109. Rosen, M.G. (1990). *Management of Labor: Physician Judgment and Patient Care.* (New York: Elsevier)

110. Gee, H. and Olah, K.S. (1988). Failure to progress in labour. In Studd, J. (ed.) *Progress in Obstetrics and Gynaecology*, vol. 10, pp. 159–82. (Edinburgh: Churchill-Livingstone)

111. O'Driscoll, K., Foley, M. and MacDonald, D. (1984). Active management of labor as an alternative to cesarean section for dystocia. *Obstet. Gynecol.*, **63**, 485–90

112. Phillips, R.D. and Freeman, M. (1974). The management of the persistant occiput posterior position: a review of 552 consecutive cases. *Obstet. Gynecol.*, **43**, 171–7

113. Philpott, R.H. (1982). The recognition of cephalopelvic disproportion. *Clin. Obstet. Gynaecol.*, **9**, 609–24

114. O'Leary, J.A. (1992). *Shoulder Dystocia and Birth Injury*. (New York: McGraw-Hill, Inc.)

115. Hofmeyr, G.J. (1989). Suspected fetopelvic disproportion. In Chalmers, I., Eukin, M. and Keirse, M.J.N.C. (eds.) *Effective Care in Pregnancy and Childbirth*, pp. 493–8. (Oxford: Oxford University Press)

116. Friedman, E.A., Acker, D.B. and Sachs, B.P. (1987). *Obstetrical Decision Making*, 2nd edn., pp. 240–1. (Philadelphia: B.C. Decker Inc.)

117. Bottoms, S.F., Hirsch, V.J. and Sokol, R.J. (1987). Medical management of arrest disorders of labor: a current overview. *Am. J. Obstet. Gynecol.*, **156**, 935–9

118. Bowes, W.A. Jr (1989). Clinical aspects of normal and abnormal labor. In Creasy, R.K. and Resnik, R. (eds.) *Maternal–Fetal Medicine: Principles and Practice*, 2nd edn., pp. 510–46. (Philadelphia: W. B. Saunders)

119. Davidson, A.C., Weaver, J.B. and Davies, P. (1976). The relation between ease of forceps delivery and speed of cervical dilation. *Br. J. Obstet. Gynaecol.*, **83**, 279–83

120. Naegele, F.C. (1991). *The Obliquely Contracted Pelvis. The Classics of Obstetrics and Gynecology Library*, p. 370. (Birmingham, Alabama: Gryphon Editions)

121. Dennen, P.C. (1989). *Dennen's Forceps Deliveries*, 3rd edn. (Philadelphia: F.A. Davis Company)

122. Crichton, D. (1974). A reliable method of establishing the level of the fetal head in obstetrics. *S. Afr. Med. J.*, **48**, 784–7

123. Hillis, D.S. (1938). Diagnosis of contracted pelvis. *Ilinois Med. J.*, **74**, 131–4

124. Compton, A.A. (1990). Avoiding difficult vaginal deliveries. In Dilts, P.V. Jr and Sciarra, J.J. (eds.) *Gynecology and Obstetrics*, vol. 2, Chapter 74, pp. 1–8. (Philadelphia: J.B. Lippincott Company)

125. Parsons, M.T. and Spellacy, W.N. (1985). Prospective randomized study of X-ray pelvimetry in the primigravida. *Obstet. Gynecol.*, **66**, 76–9

126. Rayburn, W.F., Siemers, K.H. and Legino, L.J. (1989). Dystocia in late labor: determining fetal position by clinical and ultrasonic techniques. *Am. J. Perinatol.*, **6**, 316–9

127. O'Driscoll, K., Meagher, D. and Boylan, P. (1993). *Active Management of Labor*, 3rd edn. (Aylesbury: Mosby Yearbook Europe Limited)

128. Hauth, J.C., Hankins, G.G., Gilstrap, L.C., 3rd, Strikland, D.M. and Vance, P. (1986). Uterine contraction pressures with oxytocin induction/augmentation. *Obstet. Gynecol.*, **68**, 305–9

129. Kuit, J.A., Huikeshoven, F.J., Eppinga, H.G. and Wallenburg, H.G.S. (1990). A randomized comparative clinical study of soft cup and hard cup vacuum extraction. *New Tijdschr. Obstet. Gynecol.*, **103**, 289–90

Close adherence to technique dictated by sound instrument operations is of the same critical importance as is the correct perspective. Patient selection and site preparation rank as the first break and distraction of the fracture effort are the major components of technique that assure both safety and success. Unfortunately, clinicians are likely to conclude otherwise from the apparent ease of the instrument's use. This has the unfortunate tendency to promote a casual approach towards vacuum technique.

III

Vacuum extraction operations

There are many who believe it an easy matter to deliver a Woman, because Women usually practice it. In effect, there is no great Mystery when all things come right and well: But when they come wrong and contrary to Nature, it is certain that it is the most difficult and laborious of all Chirurgical Operations . . .

François Mauriceau (1637–1709)
Traité des Maladies des Femmes Grosses, 1683[1]

The literature is already replete with grisly accounts of sloughing scalps, intracranial haemorrhages, cephalhaematomata, depressed fracture of the skull, death and destruction which accord ill with our own experience . . . of the instrument (ventouse). All this has helped to fan the prejudice of reactionary obstetricians, some of whom argued fiercely with me and with apparent intelligence and then finally confessed they had never seen the instrument used or had certainly not attempted to use it themselves. Tradition dies hard and midwives of both sexes are often remarkable for their conservatism.

I. Donald
Practical Obstetric Problems, 1979[2]

III.1 OVERVIEW

Close attention to technique utilized in vacuum extraction operations is of the same critical importance as it is in forceps procedures. Patient selection, accurate cup application to the fetal head, and direction of the tractive effort are the major components of technique that assure both safety and success. Unfortunately, clinicians are likely to conclude otherwise from the apparent ease of the instrument's use. This has the unfortunate tendency to promote a casual approach towards vacuum technique.

There are additional concerns. Detailed instruction in correct vacuum extractor use is often limited to individuals in training programs that use the device. Practicing clinicians usually develop their skills by reading and self-education with direct instruction from a colleague who may or may not have fully mastered the technique. Adequate training in all vaginal operative procedures, including vacuum extraction operations, remains a serious and unsolved issue discussed in greater detail elsewhere in the text (see Chapter II, Instruments, indications, and issues, Section 3.4, Training deficiencies).

III.2 TECHNIQUE

Regardless of the vacuum extractor chosen, the basic application technique is the same (Table III.1). With the patient prepared for delivery, a pelvic examination is performed. The position, station, and attitude of the fetal head are verified. The degree of maternal discomfort is judged and anesthesia/analgesia administered, as required. If the proposed procedure has not been discussed with the patient or family, or if plans have changed following the pelvic examination, the contemplated procedure is again reviewed briefly. This not only informs the assistants of the operator's intentions, but also forces the surgeon to reformulate, condense, and briefly explain his or her intentions in an organized and simple manner.

Once an instrument has been chosen, a 'ghost' or phantom application of the vacuum extractor is performed *prior* to the attempt at cup insertion (Figure III.1). *In ghosting, the surgeon holds the vacuum cup in front of the perineum in the same angle and position expected once the extractor has been applied correctly to the fetal head.* The practitioner then rethinks the indications for the proposed procedure and mentally reviews the application and the anticipated operation. This is exactly parallel to the ghosting procedure routinely followed for forceps operations[3,4]. Regardless of the operator's experience, or the speed dictated by the clinical setting, *the ghosting step is never omitted.* The phantom application serves as an additional check on fetal position and station, establishes the correct instrument orientation, and demands that the surgeon review his or her proposed procedure[3,5].

After ghosting, the operator checks the function of the vacuum pump, attaches the vacuum hose, and enlists the aid of the assistant(s). The cup is lubricated with surgical soap or sterile lubricant. If the cup is plastic, it

Table III.1 Prerequisites for vacuum extraction operations

(1) Informed consent
(2) Cephalic presentation fetus; standard obstetric indication for instrumental delivery
(3) Occipital, midline application of vacuum cup; centered over the cranial pivot or flexing point (see Table III.2, Figures III.5 and III.6)
(4) Analgesia (if required):
       pudendal nerve block
       saddle block
       epidural anesthesia
       (rarely) general anesthesia*
(5) Operator confirmation of fetal station and position: repeat pelvic examination to establish the station, position, and deflection of the fetal head just prior to the attempted procedure
(6) Empty maternal bladder (Credé, recent voiding or catheterization)
(7) Full cervical dilation
(8) Ruptured membranes
(9) Operator decision to abandon the operation if it does not progress easily

*Not recommended

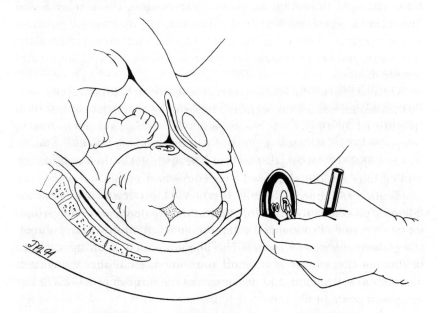

Figure III.1 Ghosting or phantom application of a metal cup extractor (Bird's cup). Left occiput position, transverse (LOT) outlet vacuum extraction. The vacuum hose is not depicted in this illustration

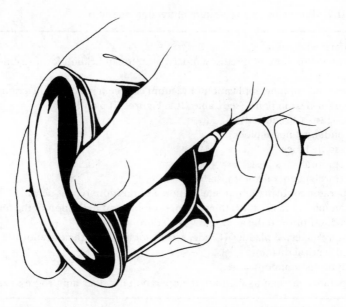

Figure III.2 A soft cup vacuum extractor (Mityvac Lined™ Vacuum Extractor, Model No. 010M, Neward Enterprises, Inc., Cucamongo, CA) is collapsed by the surgeon just prior to cup insertion

is partially collapsed by the operator's hand and introduced through the labia until it lies against the fetal head (Figure III.2). Rigid metal cups are turned sideways, the labia are gently spread, and the device slipped into the vagina (Figure III.3). Once the surgeon is certain that all maternal tissue has been excluded, an initial suction is applied, just sufficient to fix the device to the scalp (20 mmHg or less). Regular checks of application follow (Table III.2 and Figures III.4, III.5 A and B).

Before traction is attempted, the vacuum is released and the cup repositioned, if required, until an accurate application is achieved. When correctly placed, the vacuum cup is positioned centrally over the point of cranial flexion (Figure III.5 A, B)[6,7]. This *pivot point* is an imaginary spot in the midline of the fetal skull over the sagittal suture located approximately 6 cm posterior to the center of the anterior fontanelle or 1–2 cm anterior to the posterior fontanelle. This is precisely the same cranial landmark used in forceps operations to correctly align the plane of the shanks before traction is applied[3]. The primary vector of force through either the center of the vacuum cup or the plane of the forceps

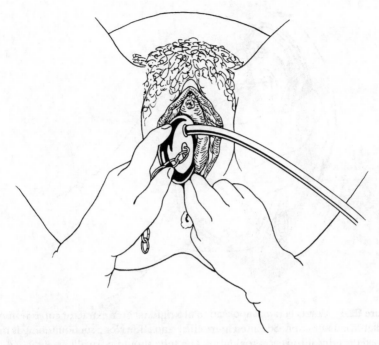

Figure III.3 Vacuum extraction operation: a Malmström/Bird vacuum extractor is inserted between the labia. Note that the suction hose is connected to the suction port *prior* to cup insertion

Table III.2 Clinical checks for correct vacuum extractor placement[3,5–7,13]

---

(1) The cup is positioned mid-sagittally with the edge of a 60 mm standard cup approximately 3 cm or two finger-breadths from the center of the anterior fontanelle (see Figure III.5)

(2) The vacuum port of the metal cup, the handle of a soft-cup extractor, or the Kobayashi blue line is directed to parallel the sagittal suture (see Figure III.1)

(3) No maternal tissue is included under the cup margin

---

shanks is directed at this point (Figure III.5). When correctly positioned, the *edge* of a standard 60 mm cup lies approximately 3 cm or two finger-breadths behind the center of the anterior fontanelle in the midline over the sagittal suture. Thus, in vacuum extraction operations the *anterior fontanelle* becomes the reference point for checking instrument

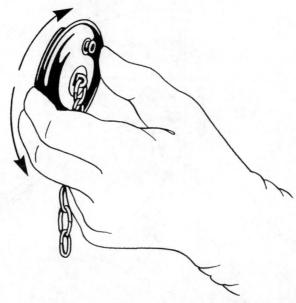

Figure III.4 Correct cranial application of a rigid vacuum extractor cup is verified by digital examination. See also Figures III.5 and III.6. Note: suction tubing is not depicted in this illustration for clarity. The tube should normally be attached to the vacuum port *prior* to cup insertion

application. Access to the posterior fontanelle is partially or completely blocked once the extractor cup is in place, rendering this familiar landmark unusable.

The physics for the use of force in vacuum extraction parallels that for classic forceps operations. The critical checks for confirming correct application of both the vacuum extractor and forceps are necessary as the safety and success of the operation depend upon maintaining cranial flexion during the extraction. Cranial flexion presents the smallest possible diameter of the presenting part to the birth canal[3,6,7]. The cranial flexion (as opposed to extension) also limits distortion, thus minimizing the risks of intracranial injury as traction is applied, avoiding excessive tension on the falx/tentorium (Figure III.6). To apply traction safely, several other points are important. The pull must be oriented along the midline of the sagittal suture. This avoids an oblique traction on the fetal head, which of itself may increase the work of extraction and predispose to failure[8,9]. In order to follow cranial rotation, either the handle of a disposable vacuum cup, the blue line of the Kobayashi device, or the vacuum port of the

(A)

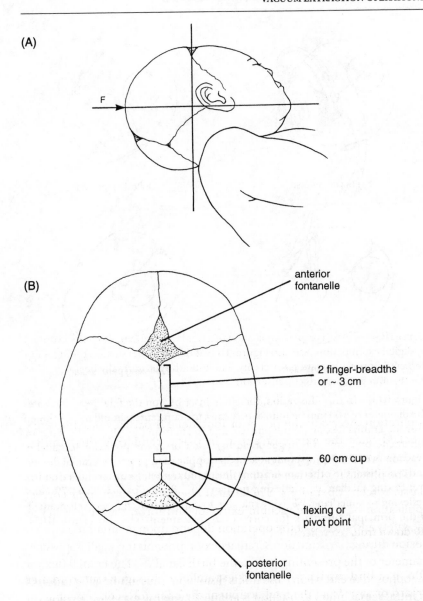

(B)

anterior
fontanelle

2 finger-breadths
or ~ 3 cm

60 cm cup

flexing or
pivot point

posterior
fontanelle

Figure III.5 (A) As illustrated, the *flexing* or *pivot point* (**F**) of the fetal head is located mid-sagitally, approximately 6 cm from the center of the anterior fontanelle or 2 cm in advance of the posterior fontanelle. When a standard vacuum cup is applied, the *cup edge* will lie approximately 3 cm or two finger-breadths behind the *anterior fontanelle*. The posterior fontanelle is often covered by a correctly applied cup and is thus not useful as a landmark. (B) This indicates the same site as viewed from above. Traction centered over this site promotes cranial flexion (see also Figure III.6)

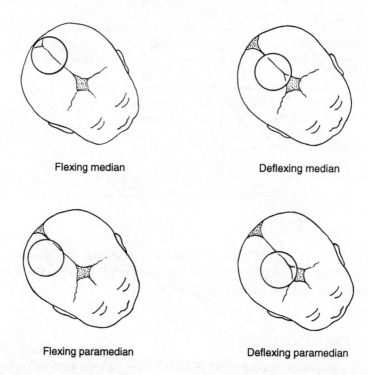

Flexing median   Deflexing median

Flexing paramedian   Deflexing paramedian

Figure III.6 In this illustration, the circle inscribed on the fetal head indicates the diameter of a 60 mm vacuum cup. Ideally, the cup center should be positioned over the cranial flexing point approximately 6 cm from the edge of the anterior fontanelle or 2 cm (two finger-breadths) anterior to the posterior fontanelle. Traction over the flexing point in a median application promotes cranial flexion and synclitism; the other applications illustrated do not. Extraction failure rates are: flexing median 4%, deflexing median 29%, flexing paramedian 17%, and deflexing paramedian 35%. Note that due to cup position the *anterior* fontanelle is the principal landmark for correct cup placement (see also Figure III.5). (Redrawn from reference 6)

O'Neil or Bird cup is positioned to lie parallel to the sagittal suture, either toward or away from the fetal occiput at the operator's convenience.

The apparent ease of vacuum extraction application tends to lull the inexperienced operator into assuming that any size cup or any location on the fetal scalp is equally satisfactory. This is not so. The smaller the cup, the greater the shear force to the scalp edge and thus the higher the possibility of soft tissue injury[10]. Also, in comparison to larger diameter devices, smaller cups require higher vacuum to maintain the same traction

Table III.3 Vacuum conversion table

mmHg	inches Hg	lb/in²	kg/cm²
760	29.9	14.7	1.03
700	27.9	13.5	0.95
600	23.6	11.6	0.82
500	19.7	9.7	0.68
400	15.7	7.7	0.54
300	11.8	5.8	0.41
200	7.9	3.9	0.27
100	3.9	1.9	0.13

force. Thus, while rigid metal Malmström/Bird and O'Neil cup sets include a small size cup and smaller cup sizes are provided by the major soft cup manufacturers, they should not be used.

III.3 TRACTION

Once a correct cup application is established, full vacuum is applied (0.8 kg/cm², 550–600 mmHg, 11.6 lb/in²). When a soft (Kobayashi or other plastic extractor) cup is used, the vacuum may be promptly raised to 0.8 kg/cm² (550–600 mmHg) by an electric or hand pump. If a Bird, O'Neil, or Malmström rigid cup has been applied, it has been traditionally taught that the vacuum is best raised by 0.2 kg/cm² every 2 min until the working pressure of 0.8 kg/cm² is generated. Alternatively, recent recommendations for rigid cups have been that traction may follow within 2 min of full suction without further waiting for the development of a chignon[6,11]. For appropriate vacuum pressures, please see Table III.3.

The pull must follow a specific vector of force, mimicking the normal pelvic curve (Figure III.7). Depending upon the station of the fetal head, the angle for the vector of force varies considerably and the operator may have to undergo substantial gymnastics in order to apply traction in the direction required. An episiotomy is performed, if necessary, when the posterior perineum bulges or if maternal soft tissue impedes the easy descent of the presenting part (see Chapter IV, Complications and birth injuries, Section 3, Maternal injuries). The higher the presenting part, the lower the extractor handle must be and the greater the requirement

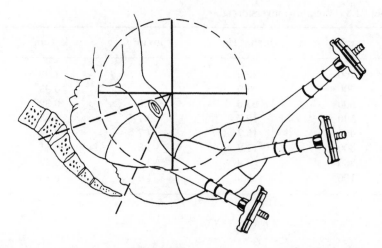

Figure III.7   The course of the fetal head and the required vector of traction as the fetal head descends through the pelvic curve (Carus' curve) during a vacuum extraction operation using a silastic vacuum extractor (Kobayashi instrument). The patient is in dorsal lithotomy postion. Note that as the fetal station changes so does the required vector of traction

for early episiotomy. As the head crowns, a Ritgen maneuver secures the chin (Figure III.8). The vacuum is then released, the cup is removed and the delivery completed.

Traction efforts are timed to coincide with uterine contractions, as they are in a forceps operation. During the extraction operation, tension is allowed to build gradually, paralleling the uterine contractions. As each contraction wanes, the tension on the extractor handle is progressively relaxed. At the surgeon's discretion, the vacuum can either be maintained or reduced to ≤ 200 mmHg (0.2 kg/cm^2) between contractions.

A rigid metal cup should be applied to the scalp under maximal suction for no more than 20–25 min. Ideally, the vacuum should be released between traction efforts. If the procedure requires more than three to four pulls reconsideration is necessary. Prolonged extraction times increase the risk of fetal scalp injury and may increase the likelihood for intracranial hemorrhage.

Time limits for plastic or soft cup applications are not established. Nonetheless, when one of these instruments is chosen, it is prudent not to exceed the same 20–25 min limit, although risk of scalp injury is arguably lower with soft than with the rigid metal cups. Twenty minutes is

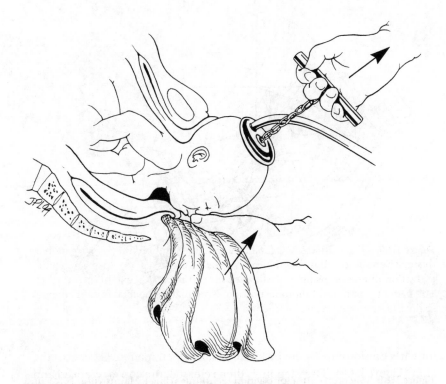

Figure III.8 Modified Ritgen maneuver and perineal management during a vacuum extraction operation using a Malmström/Bird vacuum extractor. The cup and chain assume a near 90° angle to the birth canal as the head extends

ample time for four or more traction efforts[12]. Independent of time considerations, prompt re-evaluation of the procedure is mandatory if the child has not been delivered after four traction efforts[3,13].

During traction, the best technique for the surgeon is to place the non-dominant hand within the vagina, palpating the fetal scalp with one finger and placing the thumb and remaining fingers on the extractor cup to gauge the relative position of the cup edge to the scalp (Figure III.9)[7,14–16]. So positioned, the clinician follows the descent of the presenting part and can better judge the appropriate angle for traction while detecting early cup separation. *The bimanual technique reduces the risk of sudden cup displacement and should be used with all types of vacuum extractors.* If the pull is oblique, digital traction against the cup may also reduce the

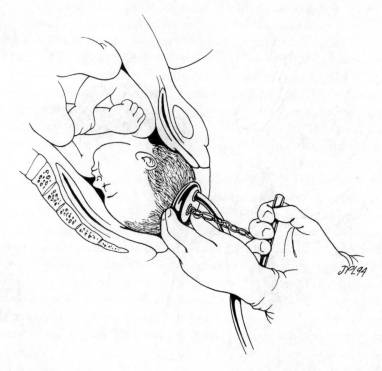

Figure III.9 Vacuum extractor traction technique using a Malmström/Bird cup applied to a fetal head in the occiput anterior (OA) position is illustrated. Note position of the operator's fingers for the vaginal hand as traction is applied

possibility of displacement for rigid metal cups and potentially for plastic extractors as well.

Incorrectly oriented traction efforts are a common problem and the usual cause of extraction failure. In vacuum extraction, as in unassisted parturition, the presenting part descends by overcoming maternal soft tissue resistance, while cranial rotation occurs spontaneously. If the vector of force applied by the operator is angled either too anteriorly or too posteriorly, descent is difficult or impossible and the likelihood of maternal or fetal injury is increased. If traction is oriented too *anteriorly*, the operation fails as the vacuum extractor pulls against the unyielding resistance of the bony pelvis. Alternatively, a pull oriented too *posteriorly* is also unsuccessful or difficult because of soft tissue resistance and the risk of maternal perineal injury.

Descent must begin with the first traction effort. Failure to make station with the presenting part as traction is applied requires immediate reassessment[5,7]. Clinicians must avoid repetitive trials of what Bird terms *negative traction*[15]. This is traction that draws the fetal scalp away from the skull but fails to result in descent of the skull. Negative traction is believed to result in rapid pressure fluctuations within the fetal cranium, potentially avulsing bridging veins. This *may* predispose to potentially serious intracranial and/or scalp hemorrhage. If the fetal head does not advance with the first pull, there is a reason. The prudent practitioner must seek it out immediately.

It is important to re-emphasize the importance of judgment and forbearance in trials of vaginal instrumental delivery. Incorrect cup placement or poorly directed traction efforts are the cause for most failed vacuum operations. Poor vacuum traction technique also predisposes to fetal injury. An unsuccessful vacuum extraction operation delays delivery, possibly contributing to fetal asphyxia/hypoxia. Finally, failure also tempts the imprudent surgeon to entertain performing a potentially traumatic forceps operation in a setting of possible (or probable) cephalo–pelvic disproportion[5,17] (see discussion of trial operations, Chapter II, Instruments, indications, and issues, Section 2.4, Trials of instrumental delivery).

3.1 Occiput anterior positions

Any of the available vacuum extractors can be applied in occiput anterior positions (OA, LOA, ROA). Standard application and traction technique is used as previously described. The indications for such procedures are the same as those for forceps operations at similar station.

3.2 Occiput posterior and occiput transverse positions

Occiput posterior (OP, LOP, ROP) and asynclitic occiput transverse (OT, LOT, ROT) positions are special cases. Vacuum extraction is often difficult in OP or OT applications due to problems in applying the cup correctly to the usually deflexed fetal head[7,15,18,19]. A disadvantage of both the Kobayashi and the popular design plastic disposable extractors is that their long, relatively rigid shafts function like inflexible rods. Their cups are difficult to position correctly when the fetal occiput is posterior or the fetal head is deflexed as the perineal soft tissue precludes a correct application. Thus, in experienced hands, forceps are often more useful in OP presentations involving cranial deflection, unless a special 'OP' metal or plastic cup is available. Recent trials of new soft cup vacuum extractors such as the Mityvac 'M'™ Cup suggest that there is a role for these plastic vacuum cups in selected OT or OP presentations when the fetal head is minimally deflexed[20]. In general, an OP vacuum extraction is more difficult than is an anterior or transverse presentation and the likelihood of failure correspondingly greater[21].

3.3 Positions requiring rotation

Vacuum extraction technique is the same for cranial positioning that classically require instrumental rotation (ROA, LOA, LOT, ROT, etc.). The cup is applied in the usual fashion, the standard checks made, and traction applied. The fetal head will spontaneously rotate as the presenting part descends. Some operators assist this spontaneous rotation by accompanying the vacuum extraction with digitally applied cranial pressure to *gently* direct the head in the correct direction. However, this is usually unnecessary and may prove counter-productive. Attempts to rotate the vacuum cup are usually to no avail and this procedure is *not* recommended. Cup rotation usually just promotes cup displacement and if performed with a rigid metal cup may promote scalp laceration. Cranial rotation will occur as the fetal head follows the normal mechanism of descent, assisted by the combined efforts of the woman (in expulsion) and the surgeon (in traction).

3.4 Special applications

Application of the vacuum extractor at high station or without full cervical dilation is *contraindicated*. However, fetal distress at advanced dilation or the extraction of a second twin are possible exceptions under special, limited circumstances, by experienced clinicians. When fetal distress occurs in a multiparous patient with an adequate pelvis and advanced cervical dilation, vacuum extraction may be attempted to expedite delivery as soon as the fetal head engages. The patient is instructed to push with contractions while *simultaneous* preparations for Cesarean delivery are made by delivery personnel *other than the vaginal surgeon*. If the extraction does not progress promptly, or if an adequate number of assistants are not available, a Cesarean is performed as soon as the necessary surgical preparations are completed.

If prompt delivery of a second twin is required, often the head can be grasped with the vacuum extractor as engagement occurs. The subsequent extraction is usually easy given the existing advanced cervical dilation and soft tissue relaxation that follow delivery of the first infant. Concomitant real-time ultrasound scanning assists the surgeon in guiding the fetal head into the pelvis, assures proper cranial flexion, and monitors fetal heart rate. Such procedures are not for the inexperienced obstetric surgeon and should be attempted only when adequately trained personnel are present to perform Cesarean delivery or version and extraction if the procedure does not proceed easily (see Chapter II, Instruments, indications, and issues, Section 2.2.3, Presumed fetal jeopardy/fetal distress).

REFERENCES

1. Mauriceau, F. (1663). In Hugh Chamberlen (ed.) *Traité des Maladies des Femmes Grosses*, 2nd edn., p. 204

2. Donald, I. (1979). *Practical Obstetric Problems*, 5th edn., p677. (London: Lloyd-Luke)

3. O'Grady, J.P. (1988). *Modern Instrumental Delivery*. (Baltimore: Williams & Wilkins)

4. Dennen, P.C. (1989). *Dennen's Forceps Deliveries*, 3rd edn. (Philadelphia: F.A. Davis Company)

5. O'Grady, J.P. and Gimovsky, M. (1993). Instrumental delivery: a lost art? In Studd (ed.) *Progress in Obstetrics and Gynaecology*, vol. 10, pp. 183–212. (New York: Churchill-Livingstone)

6. Vacca, A. (1990). The place of the vacuum extractor in modern obstetric practice. *Fet. Med. Rev.*, **2**, 103–22

7. Vacca, A. (1992). *Handbook of Vacuum Extraction in Obstetric Practice*. (London: Edward Arnold)

8. Vacca, A. (1993). Letter to the editor. Effect of angular traction on the performance of modern vacuum extractors. *Am. J. Obstet. Gynecol.*, **169**, 748–9

9. Muise, K.L., Duchon, M.A. and Brown, R.H. (1992). Effect of angular traction on the performance of modern vacuum extractors. *Am. J. Obstet. Gynecol.*, **167**, 1125–9

10. Duchon, M.A., De Murd, N.A. and Brown, R.H. (1988). Laboratory comparison of modern vacuum extractors. *Obstet. Gynecol.*, **71**, 155–8

11. Svenningsen, L. (1987). Birth progression and traction forces developed under vacuum extraction after slow or rapid application of suction. *Eur. J. Obstet. Gynecol. Reprod. Biol.*, **26**, 105–12

12. Ngan, H.Y.S., Tang, G.W.K. and Ma, H.K. (1986). Vacuum extractor: a safe instrument? *Aust. NZ J. Obstet. Gynaecol.*, **26**, 177–81

13. Laufe, L.E. and Berkus, M.D. (1992). *Assisted Vaginal Delivery*. (New York: McGraw-Hill Inc.)

14. Malmström, T. and Jansson, I. (1965). Use of the vacuum extractor. *Clin. Obstet. Gynaecol.*, **8**, 893–913

15. Bird, G.C. (1976). The importance of flexion in vacuum extractor delivery. *Br. J. Obstet. Gynaecol.*, **83**, 194–200

16. Bird, G.C. (1982). The use of the vacuum extractor. *Clin. Obstet. Gynaecol.*, **9**, 641–61

17. Pelosi, M.A. and Pelosi, M.A. III (1992). Letter to the Editor. A randomized comparison of assisted vaginal delivery by obstetric forceps and polyethylene vacuum cup. *Obstet. Gynecol.*, **79**, 638–9

18. Cohn, M., Barclay, C., Fraser, R., Zaklama, M., Johanson, R., Anderson, D. and Walker, C. (1989). A multicentre randomised trial comparing delivery with a silicone rubber cup and rigid metal vacuum extractor cups. *Br. J. Obstet. Gynaecol.*, **96**, 545–51

19. Hammarström, M., Csemiczky, G. and Belfrage, P. (1986). Comparison between the conventional Malmström extractor and a new extractor with silastic cup. *Acta. Obstet. Gynecol. Scand.*, **65**, 791–2

20. Ross, M.G. (1994). Vacuum delivery by soft cup extraction. *Contemp. Ob./Gyn.*, **39**, 48–53

21. Johanson, R., Pusey, J., Livera, N. and Jones, P. (1989). North Staffordshire/Wigan assisted delivery trial. *Br. J. Obstet. Gynaecol.*, **96**, 537–44

IV

Complications and birth injuries

These signatures may teach midwives patience, and persuade them to let nature alone to perform her own worke, and not to disquiet women by their strugglings, for such enforcements rather hinder the birthe than any waie promote it.

Percivall Willughby (1596–1685)
Observations in Midwifery, 1670[1]

Obstetrics is not one of the exact sciences, and in our penury of truth we ought to be accurate in our statements, generous in our doubts, tolerant in our convictions . . .

James Young Simpson (1811–1870)[2]

IV.1 RISKS: AN OVERVIEW

Vacuum extraction is not without risks. Most are inconsequential but serious injuries are possible. Risks for injury are both maternal and fetal. During vacuum-assisted delivery, direct injuries to the fetal scalp or cranium arise from the effects of traction. The large majority of such lesions are mild scalp abrasions. Nonetheless, more serious and even fatal fetal cranial injuries are also possible, albeit markedly uncommon[3,5–12]. Maternal injuries occur due to episiotomy extensions or birth canal lacerations, as may complicate any instrumental delivery (Table IV.1).

Mechanical injuries to mother and infant from vacuum extraction are largely but not invariably avoidable by strict adherence to technique. However, the avoidance of *all* injuries is a difficult proposition. Some problems arise in the application of instruments in complex cases which involve difficult judgments, especially the initial decision to attempt a vaginal extraction operation. In such settings, although the vaginal route appears best and the vacuum instrument is properly utilized, injury results simply because of inappropriate case selection. Injury can also result from delays in definitive treatment of fetal jeopardy/fetal distress, or result from various unforeseen obstetric or neonatal complications (e.g. pelvic fasciitis or a hemorrhage associated with a pre-existing fetal coagulopathy).

Experience and the natural reserve and caution of the obstetric surgeon reduces the risks inherent in extraction operations. As long as recurrent cup displacement does not occur and operators are careful

Table IV.1   Potential complications associated with vacuum extraction operations

Maternal

Direct
Episiotomy extension: sphincter tears, extension into the rectal mucosa
Soft tissue injuries: lacerations or ecchymosis of cervix, vaginal wall,
para-urethral tissues
Hemorrhage, uterine atony

Indirect
Fistula formation: vesico or rectovaginal
Infection: laceration/episiotomy/urinary tract
Bladder or rectal sphincter dysfunction

Fetal

Direct
Scalp injury: lacerations, abrasions, ecchymoses, necrosis
Cephalhematoma
Subgaleal (subaponeurotic) hematoma
Skull fracture, disruption of sutures
Intracranial hemorrhage (parenchymal, subdural, intraventricular,
subarachnoid)
Other soft tissue injuries
Nerve injuries
Exsanguination

Indirect
Anemia, hyperbilirubinemia
Shoulder dystocia: Erb/Duchenne, Klumpke or Weigart palsy,
clavicular or long bone fracture
Low Apgar scores, meconium aspiration
Infection
Leptomeningeal cysts
Scalp infection/abscess

with traction technique, most infant injuries from vacuum extraction are of trivial consequence. Operator attention to properly directed traction efforts will similarly obviate many but not all maternal injuries. In order to minimize the risks of injury, accoucheurs must strongly resist excess of effort as well as inappropriate case selection by close adherence to protocol.

In the following sections, specific maternal and fetal injuries are discussed. In modern practice, any difficulty with vaginal delivery should inspire immediate caution in the surgeon rather than a determination to prevail. The obstetrician can easily overpower the fetus in any vaginal instrumental delivery but the costs can (and usually do) prove unacceptable!

IV.2 FETAL INJURIES

2.1 Chignon and minor scalp injuries

Diagnosis

The chignon is easily identified by direct observation as an area of localized scalp edema molded to the shape of the extractor cup. This localized caput is given a characteristic 'plateau' configuration by the effects of the vacuum. Other scalp injuries such as abrasions and ecchymosis are similarly diagnosed by direct observation (Figures IV.1 and IV.2).

Incidence

Some extent of chignon formation accompanies all vacuum extraction operations. In a review of 3543 extractions performed with the Malmström metal cup, Plauché[8] reported a 12.6% mean incidence of minor scalp trauma. Scalp injuries, including the chignon, occur with less frequency when soft cup extractors are used, but reliable incidence figures are not available[7,12,13].

Comments

Most scalp abrasions and ecchymoses following vacuum extraction are of little clinical importance[7]. Serious scalp injuries including lacerations or

(A)

(B)

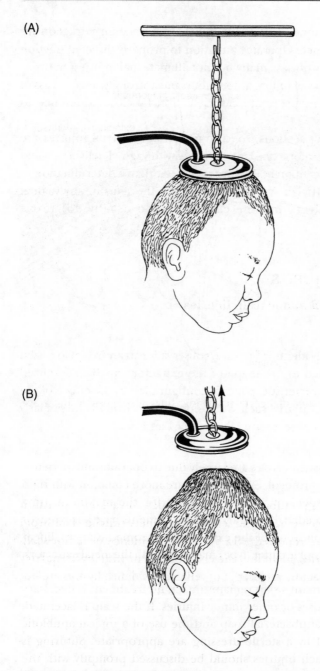

Figure IV.1   (A) Rigid vacuum extraction cup application (Bird cup depicted) and (B) resultant chignon. See text for discussion and details

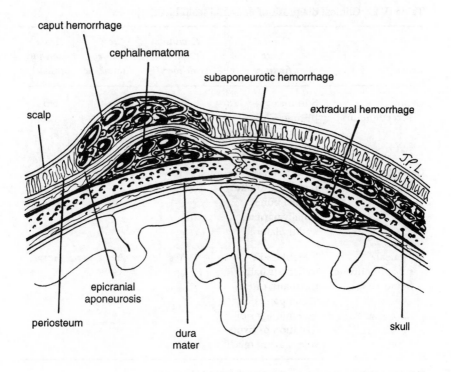

caput hemorrhage

cephalhematoma

subaponeurotic hemorrhage

extradural hemorrhage

scalp

epicranial
aponeurosis

periosteum

dura
mater

skull

Figure IV.2 Cross-section of the fetal scalp indicating sites of possible injury. See text for details

localized skin or tissue necrosis are largely due to operator inexperience or failure to follow protocol. Such injuries are more common with rigid cup extractors, especially when guidelines for the maximum time application are exceeded, if several cup displacements have occurred, or if there was malapplication of the extractor[7,8]. In some instances, linear scalp lacerations ('cookie cutter' type) may occur with the metal extractors, albeit rarely.

As long as the infant's skin remains intact, no treatment is necessary for simple ecchymoses or other minor injuries. If the scalp is lacerated, cleansing with an antibacterial soap and the use of a topical antibiotic ointment followed by a sterile dressing are appropriate. Suturing is required rarely. Such injuries should be discussed promptly with the parents and pediatrician to avoid any undue anxiety or a potentially uncomfortable situation. Extensive scalp lesions should be carefully

Table IV.2 Clinical diagnosis of neonatal scalp birth injuries[9,16]

Lesion	Clinical scalp findings	Expansion post-delivery?	Cross suture lines?	Acute hemorrhage possible?
Caput succedaneum	Soft mass, pitting, commonly midline, over vertex	No	Yes	No
Cephal-hematoma*	Firm to tense, restricted to one cranial bone, usually parietal and unilateral	Yes	No	No
Subgaleal/ subaponeurotic[†] hemorrhage	Variable, soft to firm, usually fluctuant, often accompanied by systemic signs of irritation or hypo-volemia/anemia	Yes	Yes	Yes

*Underlying skull fracture may be present in 10–35% of cases
†May be accompanied by a coagulation defect and/or cardiovascular collapse

evaluated to exclude underlying skull fractures, cephalhematomas or other serious intracranial injuries (Table IV.2)[3,7-9,11].

The chignon itself is less an injury than an accentuation of the normal process of caput formation and usually disappears within 12–24 h. The formation of a chignon of some degree is an unavoidable part of vacuum extraction but is more common with the rigid metal extractors. The significance of the chignon originates with the reaction it elicits from the pediatrician and the family. The chignon contributed to the initial slow acceptance of vacuum extraction in American practice because it is unusual and even frightening to the uninitiated.

More serious scalp injuries are possible. These uncommon lesions include partial scalp necrosis, subcutaneous emphysema and the formation of cephalhematomas and subaponeurotic (subgaleal) hematomas (see Table IV.2)[6,7,14,15].

2.2   Cephalhematoma

Diagnosis

A cephalhematoma is a blood collection that lies beneath the pericranium, and arises from the laceration of subperiosteal vessels[16]. On physical examination, a soft-to-firm well-circumscribed cranial swelling that *does not move with the scalp* is palpated. Immediately following delivery, large cephalhematomas may be difficult to distinguish clinically from the normal caput succedaneum. Table IV.2 outlines the principal clinical differences between the major scalp lesions.

Incidence

Cephalhematomas occur more frequently in instrumental than in spontaneous deliveries, especially following mid-forceps operations and vacuum extraction procedures (Table IV.3)[13,17-35]. The mean incidence is 5.5%[8] although many of the reported cases in these series were in association with rigid metal extractors.

Comment

Cephalhematomas are contrasted with caput succedaneum and subaponeurotic hemorrhages. In caput succedaneum, the scalp effusion is entirely independent of the periosteum of the bone and consists of edema. The swelling of caput is moderately firm and does not shift dependently. It can cover a substantial portion of the scalp and, most importantly in diagnosis, extends across suture lines. In cephalhematomas the hemorrhage is confined in size by the limits of a single cranial bone due to the firm attachments of the periosteum at the periphery of each bony plate.

Cephalhematomas are usually inconsequential unless they conceal an underlying skull fracture which may rarely accompany a vacuum extraction[19,35-37]. Thus, if a large cephalhematoma is present following a difficult delivery, a cranial radiograph is prudent to exclude an occult skull fracture. For uncomplicated cephalhematomas, no specific therapy is required, and they normally regress spontaneously without complication. At times, the period for resolution may be as long as several

Table IV.3 Frequency of cephalhematomas reported in several series of vacuum extraction (VE) deliveries. (Modified from reference 8)

Series	No. of VE deliveries	Cephalhematomas	
		n	%
Amosy and Ahlander[17]	216	5	2.3
Zilliacus and Sjöstedt[18]	508	40	7.9
Brandstrup and Lange[19]	651	36	5.5
Mishell and Kelly[20]	25	2	8.0
Spritzer[21]	60	3	4.2
Hammerstein and Gromotke[22]	365	18	4.9
Guardino and O'Brien[23]	114	7	6.1
Munsat et al.[24]	109	28	25.9
Roskowski et al.[25]	520	31	5.95
Lasbrey et al.[26]	121	20	17.0 ('often small')
Malmström[27]	520	68	13.2
Barth & Newton[28]	100	18	18.0
Chalmers[29]	700	7	6.1 (+ 4.5% scalp effusion)
St. Vincent Buss[30]	199	11	5.5
Brat[31]	1135	27	2.4
Schenker and Serr[32]	299	12	4.0
Widen et al.[33]	201	11	5.5
Plauché[8]	228	23	10.0
Broekhuizen et al.[34]	256	10	3.9
Fahmy[35]	2670	117	4.4
Total	8998	494	Mean 5.5

weeks. Occasionally, neonatal anemia or hyperbilirubinemia results from a cephalhematoma or its subsequent resorption. These lesions are more common in prolonged extractions of larger infants especially where there have been cup displacement(s)[35]. These lesions tend to occur more often in the delivery of the nulliparous, and in association with a male fetus.

2.3 Subgaleal (subaponeurotic) hemorrhages

Diagnosis

A subgaleal hematoma is a collection of blood in the space between the periosteum of the skull (pericranium) and the galea aponeurotica (epicranial aponeurous). These hemorrhages are dangerous due to the large potential space for blood accumulation[11,16,38]. The scalp examination of most infants with subgaleal hematomas is quite characteristic. The swelling is diffuse and not fixed. It usually shifts dependently when the infant's head is repositioned. On palpation, the scalp has an unusual feel – like fluid trapped in a plastic bag – and characteristically indents easily. Subaponeurotic hematomas may also present as a swelling which is indistinguishable from scalp edema, usually over the occiput. Uncommonly, the scalp is tense or firm. Usually, in the latter case, blood loss is extensive and systemic signs of vascular collapse are also present, suggesting the correct diagnosis. On occasion, scalp discoloration from blood extravasation appears in the frontal or occipital regions.

In some instances, the cranial findings are unremarkable and hypotension and pallor are the only presenting signs. There may be associated signs of cerebral irritation, including convulsions. A history of vacuum extraction, evidence of scalp injury, a rising pulse rate, increased respiratory rate, and clinical documentation of a rapid drop in hemoglobin/hematocrit strongly suggest this lesion. The correct diagnosis can be quickly confirmed by a cranial ultrasound, which reveals a dependent, echochoic space in the scalp (see Figure IV.2 and Table IV.2).

Incidence

Approximately one-half of subgaleal hemorrhages follow vacuum extraction, and one-third are associated with spontaneous vaginal deliveries. In vacuum extraction operations the incidence is estimated to be 1/1300 procedures[6,8,11].

Comments

Subgaleal hematomas are potentially serious and differ significantly from cephalhematomas[8,9,38]. As subgaleal hemorrhages occur outside the periosteum they can rapidly extend across suture lines and large quantities

81

of blood can collect rapidly, especially if a neonatal coagulopathy exists. The concealed nature of these hemorrhages and their varying presentation make them potentially dangerous. In approximately one-half of these cases a congenital coagulopathy is a predisposing factor. Subaponeurotic hemorrhage is more frequent when the neonate's vitamin K-dependent coagulation factors (factors II, VII, IX, X) are low, or if fetal hypoxia was present at birth. Unfortunately, neonatal administration of parenteral vitamin K does not help as the increase in coagulation activity is not rapid enough to prevent the bleeding. Thus the transfusion of blood and blood products is the appropriate therapy. It is unclear why but it is likely that the incidence of subaponeurotic hemorrhage is reduced by the use of soft cup extractors. Prolonged difficult extractions and multiple vacuum cup displacements are believed to be predisposing factors[11].

Most cases are identified within the first hours of delivery. In other instances the lesion may not result in symptoms for several days. Treatment is supportive. Once the diagnosis is established, blood and blood products are transfused, vitamin K_1 (phytonadione) is administered and cardiovascular support is given as needed. Vigorous treatment may be required.

In non-fatal cases resorption of the sequestered hemoglobin often results in hyperbilirubinemia and neonatal jaundice. In a dated review, Plauché[8] reported a mortality rate of 22.8%. In modern practice with early diagnosis and prompt therapy, serious morbidity and mortality should be rare. *The important point is to suspect and treat the lesion early before serious cardiovascular collapse develops.*

Particularly if there has been a difficult vacuum extraction operation, the surgeon should alert the pediatrician to the facts of the case and of his or her concern about a possible scalp/cranial injury. This notification should be documented in the medical record either in a progress note or the dictated procedure note.

2.4 Intracranial hemorrhage

Diagnosis

Intracranial hemorrhage commonly presents as neonatal depression, apnea, and/or shock. Occasionally, increased irritability, poor feeding or convulsions are the initial symptoms. The diagnosis is suspected when such abnormal neonatal behavior accompanies an obvious cranial injury or an instrumental delivery[16]. As discussed later, the signs and symptoms of injury may be delayed until several hours postpartum and, uncommonly, even later.

Incidence

Intracranial hemorrhage is an uncommon but feared complication of vacuum extraction[3,-9,39]. The low frequency of subarachnoid, subdural, and intraparenchymal bleeds, as well as discrepancies in reporting methods between series, make it difficult to judge the actual prevalence. In collected series the incidence is reported to vary from 0.2 to 8%. The best overall estimate from the literature is approximately 0.35–0.75%, or one event for every 200 or fewer *unselected* vacuum extraction procedures[3]. However, this risk figure is likely to be too great, as much of these data were generated by reports published at a time when extractors were used in a different fashion than is currently recommended. Avoidance of heroic procedures, eschewing vacuum procedures on premature infants, and strict adherence to protocol will reduce the risk to a minimum.

Comments

While difficult vacuum extractions commonly produce scalp injuries, serious intracranial damage is most uncommon. Strict attention to appropriate indications and case selection for vacuum extraction and the use of proper technique are essential in preventing intracranial trauma. The majority of intracranial hemorrhages associated with vacuum extraction are observed in premature infants or in cases complicated by severe asphyxia. Many injuries might be avoided by more rigorous case selection. However, classic subdural hemorrhages have been described in association with both complicated and uncomplicated vacuum extraction operations in otherwise apparently normal neonates[3-5].

Subarachnoid, subdural, periventricular or intraparenchymal bleeding is possible. Subdural hemorrhages have a general association with difficult delivery[6,40,41]. In a 1987 review of 41 cases, Romodanov and Brodsky[41] reported that breech presentation, macrosomia (> 4000 g), vacuum extraction, and protracted labor are the principal clinical events associated with subdural hematomas. Such intracranial lesions are similar to those described by a prior generation of obstetricians in association with traumatic forceps operations or difficult breech extraction deliveries[42].

Subdural hemorrhages occur largely as a result of distortion of the fetal cranium during the birth process. In theory, deformation of the fetal skull with rapid second-stage labor, or from cranial traction of assisted delivery, stretches and eventually ruptures the leaves of the falx/tentorium at their fixed attachments to the cranial side-wall. The resultant subdural hemorrhage either dissects anteriorly to involve the hemispheres or extends downward into the posterior fossa[7,38].

In a test of this hypothesis, Awon[43] has described distortion of the fetal parietal bone with vacuum extractor application. It is theorized that such distortion might lead to disruption of intracranial vessels and subsequent hemorrhage. Controversy surrounds Awon's finding, however, as his studies were performed on fresh stillborns. Whether the distortions depicted in his published radiographs are reflective of what occurs in the intact, living fetus is unclear.

While vacuum extraction delivery is an extremely frequent obstetric procedure, an associated intracranial hemorrhage is at best uncommon (< 1%). While trauma is suspected in cases associated with difficult delivery, the combination of events that predispose to hemorrhage in uncomplicated cases is uncertain. As suggested above, delivery technique, prematurity, fetal condition, and case selection influence the likelihood of injury. Observations from clinical experience and a review of recently reported cases are suggestive of several important associations. Unfortunately, in the recently reported cases of vacuum extraction complicated by intracranial bleeding, full delivery data are not available[4,5].

Lahat and co-workers[3] report a case of subdural hemorrhage following a vacuum extraction of a 3700 g male fetus at 38 weeks' gestation in a case complicated by 'pre-eclamptic toxemia', hypertension, and 'fetal heart rate changes'. The initial Apgar scores were 9/10 at 1 and 5 min, respectively, and the basic laboratory work on the neonate was normal, although coagulation studies were not reported. In Hanigan's report of three cases[4], the course of the labors, the results of intrapartum electronic fetal monitoring, and difficulties encountered during parturition, if any, are incompletely documented. However, in two of his three described cases of vacuum-assisted delivery, the second stage lasted 5 min or less.

In contrast, Hall provides considerably more detail concerning one case of an unusually prolonged and presumably complicated extraction where both soft cup and rigid metal cup instruments were used[5]. It is unclear from this report how many traction efforts were attempted, how long the instruments were in place, or if one or more cup displacement(s) occurred. In any event, 110 min transpired in the delivery suite. The neonate developed both subaponeurotic and intracranial hemorrhages. There were also intermittent variable fetal heart rate (FHR) decelerations documented before the operative procedure. Additional details of the labor/delivery are unavailable.

Such examples illustrate factors which significantly increase the risk of fetal injury. Included among them are: abnormal FHR tracing, evidence of difficult extraction with an unusually prolonged time required for vacuum delivery operation, high fetal station at commencement of operation, or, paradoxically, the suggestion of a rapidly descending fetal head. Both the degree and rapidity of cranial distortion are probable contributing factors. Again, it is well to point out that in these recent reports the technique of extraction, number of traction efforts, the instrument(s) used, and the site of cup placement are not discussed in detail.

As noted above, intracranial subdural bleeding is more frequent following either spontaneous, precipitate labors or prolonged instrumental deliveries. The common factor here is likely to be fluctuations in intracranial pressure accompanying cranial deformation. Anatomic data suggest that small, asymptomatic bleeds occur as a consequence of both spontaneous and instrumental delivery more frequently than is suspected on clinical grounds alone[42]. Perhaps not suprisingly, co-existing fetal asphyxia and prematurity increase the risk for intracranial hemorrhages[6,44].

Neonatal signs and symptoms of intracranial hemorrhage are those of cerebral irritation. The clinical manifestations and the prognosis for recovery depend upon the amount of bleeding and its anatomic location as well as the presence of other fetal injuries. Infants may present with convulsions, spasticity, rigidity, photophobia, high-pitched cry, or depressed reflexes[3,8]. Occasionally, signs of central nervous system injury are delayed for 24 h or more. Neonates with late-presenting cerebral irritation exhibit non-specific clinical signs such as weak suck, respiratory distress, apnea, bulging fontanelle, and/or lethargy[5,16,45]. If an intracranial bleed is diagnosed, other acute but rare injuries such as skull fracture should be suspected. Rarely, other acute or long-term events such as leptomeningeal cyst formation may follow vacuum extraction operation cranial injuries[16,46]. Ultrasonic, magnetic resonance or radiographic studies are indicated if characteristic neurological signs and symptoms are noted or in the presence of unexplained anemia or cardiovascular collapse[3].

Treatment for a diagnosed intracranial hemorrhage is supportive, with blood transfusion as indicated. Extradural hemorrhages may require surgical drainage. Neurosurgical consultation is obtained, and any coagulopathy treated, if present.

Non-specific signs and symptoms of cerebral irritation occur with all types of intracranial bleeding, irrespective of etiology. Thus, it may be reasonably expected that pediatricians and neonatologists are familiar with the clinical manifestations of this rare complication of vacuum extraction. Nonetheless, as mentioned previously, if a difficult or complex extraction has been performed or if the neonate's initial condition is less than ideal, it is prudent for the surgeon to directly communicate his/her concerns about the risk of an intracranial hemorrhage directly to the pediatrician and document this discussion with a progress note in the medical record or in a dictated operative note. This communication will serve to alert the attending pediatrician/neonatologist that monitoring for signs of cerebral irritation is appropriate to best assure the well-being of the neonate (see Chapter V, Legal issues).

While intracranial hemorrhage is a rare complication of vacuum extraction, clinicians should recall that such lesions are possible even in apparently easy or uncomplicated procedures. Infants with characteristic signs of cranial hemorrhage, whether delivered following spontaneous precipitate labor, or a difficult vacuum extraction operation, should be evaluated rapidly. Prudent use of the vacuum extraction instrument will avoid many but not all such injuries. Close attention to vacuum extraction technique and case selection to avoid high-risk situations are the best means of prevention.

2.5   Shoulder dystocia

Diagnosis

Shoulder girdle dystocia occurs when the fetal shoulder (bisacromial diameter) attempts to enter the maternal pelvis but cannot pass below the pubic symphysis. This results because of the difference in dimensions between the fetal chest and the inlet of the maternal pelvis or due to malpresentation of the shoulders to the inlet, or due to both mechanisms.

A common but not invariable clinical observation with shoulder dystocia is cranial recoil. This 'turtle sign' is a characteristic, rapid retrograde movement of a usually cherubic-appearing fetal head following

Table IV.4 Incidence of brachial plexus injury in several large, unselected clinical series

Author	n/Total deliveries	Incidence/1000 live births
Vassalos et al.[56]	169/66 149	2.50
Tan[57]	57/90 436	0.63
Gordon et al.[58]	59/31 700	1.89
Specht[59]	11/19 314	0.57
McFarland et al.[60]	106/210 947	0.50
Total	402/418 546	Mean = 0.96

spontaneous or assisted delivery[47]. Its appearance is a distinct harbinger of trouble as subsequent tentative cranial traction is virtually always unsuccessful.

Incidence

The incidence of shoulder dystocia is approximately 5/1000 deliveries, which is probably a conservative estimate[48–54]. Only cases requiring special manipulations or resulting in neonatal injury are recorded consistently. Gonik[49] argues persuasively that the risk of infant injury is substantially greater in instances where the diagnosis is either not made and appropriate maneuvers are not performed or are performed too late.

The reported incidence of Erb's palsy, the most common of the brachial plexus nerve injuries associated with shoulder girdle dystocia or vaginal breech delivery, is 0.96/1000 live births (Table IV.4). The likelihood for a brachial plexus injury to follow a shoulder dystocia is approximately 10–15%[48]. Clinicians should note that cases of similar nerve injury are occasionally reported following fetal extractions at Cesarean delivery. It is also *rarely* possible for plexus injuries to occur *in utero*, but the incidence is unknown[49,55–60].

At delivery, the injured infant is usually found to be macrosomic, flaccid, and hypoxic or partially asphyxiated. Spontaneous delivery does not necessarily avoid the problem of dystocia. Approximately one-third of shoulder dystocia cases follow precipitate and uninstrumented second-stage labors[54]. In breech deliveries, the incidence of plexus injury is 175-fold greater than in cephalic presentations, with the lower roots more

Table IV.5   Potential procedures for delivery: shoulder dystocia[47-53,63-69]

Increase pelvic capacity: symphysiotomy

Decrease fetal bisacromial size: clavicular
    fracture/cleidotomy

Suprapubic pressure, directed obliquely
    Resnik, Rubin maneuver

Upward cranial displacement
    Hibbard maneuver

Maternal repositioning
    MacRoberts maneuver, knee-chest positioning

Fetal rotational maneuvers
    Woods corkscrew maneuver and its modifications
    extraction of the posterior arm

Instrumental delivery
    shoulder displacement by vectis blade
    Chavis maneuver
    Shute forceps application

Intrauterine replacement of fetal head by vaginal manipulation
    Zavanelli maneuver, cephalic replacement

Combined vaginal and intra-abdominal operation
    abdominal rescue procedure

likely to be injured. Brachial plexus injury is also associated with vacuum-assisted delivery. This is probably due to problems of unsuspected feto-pelvic disproportion and may reflect a bias towards attempting vacuum extraction in cases of borderline disproportion where forceps applications are considered inappropriate.

Comments

Shoulder dystocia is an obstetric emergency. Successful and atraumatic management depends upon rapid diagnosis, co-operation from the mother and the delivery attendants, and immediate use of specialized extraction techniques. There are a number of procedures or manipulations to relieve shoulder dystocia, all of which require knowledge of fetal and pelvic anatomy. They include reducing the size of the fetal thorax, repositioning the fetal shoulders to a larger pelvic diameter, or

Table IV.6 Management protocol for shoulder dystocia. (Modified from reference 65)

Progression of maneuvers	Procedure(s) [47–55,65–69]
Initial	McRoberts maneuver Oblique, suprapubic pressure (Hibbard/Resnik maneuver)

Secondary	Perform prior procedures; then attempt:
	 delivery of posterior shoulder
	  (Schwartz/Dixon maneuver)
	 corkscrew maneuver
	  (Woods maneuver)
	 shoulder abduction
	  (Rubin maneuver)
	 Shute forceps application*

Tertiary	Perform prior procedures; then attempt:
	 clavicular fracture
	 cephalic replacement
	  (Zavanelli maneuver)
	 symphysiotomy*
	 combined vaginal/abdominal
	  'rescue' procedure

*Only to be attempted by experienced practitioners

changing pelvic diameters (Tables IV.5 and IV.6). In unusually severe cases, replacement of the fetal head (Zavanelli or cephalic replacement maneuver) and combined Cesarean delivery with vaginal manipulations (abdominal rescue) have been advocated[50,53].

Gonik and colleagues[49] and Jennett and co-workers[55] have commented upon cases of brachial plexus injury where shoulder dystocia was either unrecognized and not reported, or may have occurred spontaneously *in utero*. Occasional cases of plexus injury follow Cesarean delivery or the outwardly atraumatic delivery of infants who are *not* macrosomic (i.e. $\leq$ 3500 g). There are, as well, reports of electromyography findings in infants with plexus injuries indicating that the lesion predates labor/delivery. It is unclear if lack of recognition of instances of dystocia at parturition or if actual *in utero* plexus injury explains these reports. Probably most brachial plexus injuries are due to unrecognized disproportion and occur during parturition. However, the evidence may also be fairly read to suggest that

Table IV.7 Incidence of shoulder dystocia by type of delivery and fetal weight. (Taken from reference 61, with permission)

Type of delivery	Fetal weight (g)	Incidence of shoulder dystocia	%
Vertex/vaginal	< 4000	6/7836	0.07
PSS + MPD*	< 4000	6/360	1.60
Vertex/vaginal	≥ 4000	8/638	1.20
PSS + MPD*	≥ 4000	13/56	23.0

*PSS, prolonged stage of labor; MPD, mid-pelvic delivery

at least *some* injuries occur spontaneously *in utero*. As discussed later, prediction of dystocia is problematic (see Chapter VI, Risk assessment, Section 2.4, Fetal macrosomia). Historical risk factors may help to identify some cases and the course of labor is partially predictive of difficulty in other instances. A particularly important circumstance is when poor second-stage progress accompanies mid-pelvic delivery in large infants (Table IV.7)[61].

In modern practice shoulder dystocia is rarely associated with fetal loss, but morbidity continues to be a problem[48,50]. Common associated injuries include soft tissue injuries to the fetal scalp, fractured long bones, fractured clavicle, and injuries to the brachial plexus. Prolonged efforts at delivery also contribute to depressed Apgar scores and hypoxia/asphyxia and its multiple sequalae. Among the most common of these injuries is brachial plexus damage.

The brachial plexus is a complex of nerves including the fifth, sixth, seventh, and eighth cervical and first and second thoracic nerve roots. The plexus is usually damaged by lateral traction on the fetal head in cases of shoulder dystocia or in vaginal breech delivery by downward traction on the shoulders in delivery of the aftercoming head. Plexus injury occurs less frequently during Cesarean delivery and as noted above may possibly occur *in utero*.

If the plexus is damaged, the neonate fails to move one hand or arm in a normal fashion and may have respiratory distress. The fifth and sixth cervical roots are most vulnerable in cephalic presentation deliveries. Damage to these nerves results in a Duchenne/Erb's palsy – the 'waiter's tip' deformity. The affected arm is rotated inward with extension and adduction. If the seventh and eighth and first thoracic roots are damaged, the forearm and hand are affected. In 2–3% of all brachial plexus injuries only these lower roots are damaged, and the lesion is known as Klumpke's paralysis.

Because the fifth cervical nerve root also gives rise to the phrenic nerve, respiratory difficulties may arise in some neonates with brachial plexus injuries; the combination is called Weigart's palsy. An ipsilateral Horner's syndrome with ptosis, miosis, and ophthalmos from involvement of the cervical sympathetic fibers of the first thoracic root spinal cord injuries may also accompany brachial nerve palsies. 'Pseudo-Erb's' palsy arises from certain injuries to the shoulder joint, including tearing of the capsule, fractures of the clavicle, or fracture, dislocation, or detachment of the upper humeral epiphysis. Because the neonate fails to move the involved extremity normally, nerve injury is suspected, but is ruled out on neurological/orthopedic examination.

Complete recovery from a brachial plexus injury is the rule, with 80% or more of injuries spontaneously regressing within 3–6 months. Lower-root or Klumpke's paralysis has a much poorer prognosis, with just 40% of cases completely recovering within a year[16].

Treatment in the newborn period is symptomatic with frequent range-of-motion exercises and splinting. Routine surgical exploration and attempts at repair are not indicated until it is clear that spontaneous improvement has failed to occur after 3–6 months of conservative therapy[62]. Surgical repair with axillary exploration, nerve transplantation, and microsurgical reconstruction can prove remarkably successful in selected cases.

Maternal risks also accompany shoulder dystocia, the most serious including postpartum uterine atony with accompanying hemorrhage. Birth canal lacerations and hematomas are additional problems. Rarely, injury to or rupture of the bladder or uterus are possible in cases of excessive manipulation in effecting delivery. Maternal morbidity also results if cephalic replacement and abdominal delivery are attempted.

What about the issue of prevention? Ultrasonic evaluation of the fetus is often recommended both for weight estimation and determination of various ratios between head and body[50]. Unfortunately, these measurements are difficult to obtain and their positive predictive value remains poor[48]. Recommendations for clinical management based on fetal weight estimates or various bodily ratios as calculated from ultrasonic examinations have not been validated sufficiently to serve as the *sole* basis for management decisions. Nonetheless, ultrasonic estimates of fetal weight are commonly obtained when clinical examination suggests macrosomia or the mother is diabetic. The issue is how to interpret and use these data.

If the fetus is estimated to be large, clinical pelvimetry and a discussion with the patient concerning management is prudent. A note reflecting this counseling should be made in the medical record. If clinical signs of pelvic adequacy are present and the course of labor is normal, the risk of serious dystocia is low but not entirely excluded. Whenever the possibility of dystocia is considered, some preparations are prudent, such as assuring adequate anesthesia and recruiting an experienced assistant for delivery (see also Chapter VI, Risk assessment, Section 2.4, Fetal macrosomia).

Depending upon the circumstances, the practitioner might use combinations of clinical and ultrasonic data to decide the mode of delivery, Cesarean or vaginal, with or without instrumental assistance. A study comparing the clinical utility of these approaches has never been undertaken and probably will never be performed. However, in considering these schemes, clinicians should recall that prevention of vaginal birth injury by Cesarean delivery is a reasonable option in only limited and extreme situations because, first, shoulder dystocia is difficult to predict, and second, there is a low incidence of permanent injury when and if dystocia does occur[48]. A better solution for injury reduction is to train practitioners to identify and avoid obviously difficult cases and to appropriately manage the remaining cases of dystocia when they do occur.

All clinicians must have a practiced series of procedures to relieve shoulder dystocia[9,47-54,64-69]. Prompt, skillful manipulations and co-ordinated use of moderate force will almost always succeed in atraumatic or minimally traumatic delivery, except in the most extreme of cases. Simple fundal pressure with accompanying cranial traction to overcome dystocia is associated with a high rate of complication, and must be avoided. Unless the anterior fetal shoulder is repositioned, fundal pressure simply compounds the problem by further wedging it against the pubic symphysis.

It is best to develop a fixed plan of management[66]. Help should be summoned. An immediate, generous episiotomy or an episioproctomy is usually suggested as a first step if a dystocia occurs. We favor episiotomy *if tightness of the perineal tissues impedes the clinician's efforts.* The rule of reason must apply. Incising the perineum is performed if this operation results in additional room for manipulation. In some cases in a multipara, if a lax perineum is present, episiotomy may not assist the extraction and a perineal incision is unnecessary. Various obstetric maneuvers for fetal delivery follow. Although these techniques are presented in a stepwise fashion, there is no fixed protocol to follow. No one manipulation has been proven to be markedly superior to another. We suggest attempting what we have discovered to be the easier procedures first. In our experience most cases of dystocia are managed without great difficulty. Regardless of which manipulation is first attempted, the clinician must master several of the standard procedures as success with any single maneuver cannot be assured. We have found that marked flexion of the mother's legs and thighs (McRoberts maneuver) is the easiest initial procedure and has been successful in our institution in many cases. We practice it routinely if a macrosomic infant is suspected, even prior to establishing the diagnosis of dystocia. If episiotomy, the McRoberts maneuver, and gentle cranial traction fail to displace the shoulder, other actions are necessary. Repositioning of the anterior shoulder is next performed with oblique suprapubic pressure (Hibbard/Resnik maneuver). If this fails, a Woods Screw maneuver is performed, or the posterior arm is delivered (Schwartz-Dixon maneuver). Fundal pressure is counter-productive and must not be used until the impacted shoulder is released by one of these standard maneuvers such as the 'rocking' maneuver suggested by Rubin. In this procedure, the fetal shoulders are manipulated too and fro laterally by suprapubic pressure. Thereafter, the most accessible fetal shoulder is pushed toward the anterior surface of the fetal chest, abducting the shoulders, decreasing the bisacromial diameter. O'Leary[50] has described protocols for shoulder dystocia management. An outline of a progressive management protocol including many of the standard maneuvers is presented in Table IV.6.

Clavicular fracture, the Zavanelli maneuver (cranial replacement), or combined vaginal and abdominal operative delivery (abdominal rescue), are suggested as the final procedures to be attempted in 'ultimate' cases of shoulder dystocia[50,64,65]. Unfortunately, none of these is an entirely satisfactory procedure. The clavicle is usually difficult to fracture, even with instruments[66]. The Zavanelli maneuver and abdominal rescue are heroic and their success and safety remain to be established[50,63,64]. Symphysiotomy is a well-established technique in non-Western obstetric practice for shoulder dystocia but should not be attempted by the unexperienced[67,68]. Fortunately, the extreme degree of delivery difficulty requiring such techniques is rare, at best. Shute[69] has also described successful shoulder dystocia release by the use of a parallel blade forceps application with rotation. This procedure also should not be attempted by the inexperienced clinician.

2.6 Retinal injury

Diagnosis

Retinal hemorrhages are diagnosed following direct ophthalmoscopic examination of the newborn. Mechanical retraction of the eyelids by an assistant may be required for adequate evaluation.

Incidence

There is a wide range of incidence for retinal hemorrhage in spontaneous and instrumentally assisted deliveries. There are positive associations between retinal hemorrhage, assisted delivery, and prolonged labor. The most significant factor affecting incidence is mode of delivery. The mean incidence in spontaneous deliveries is 27%[9]. The rate in forceps-delivered infants is not significantly different at 29%. Cesarean delivery appears to be protective, with a low incidence of approximately 2%. Vacuum extraction, however, increases the incidence of retinal hemorrhage to approximately 40%[71]. The period of time that vacuum force is applied to the fetus is important. The longer the duration of the extraction operation and the greater its difficulty, the greater the incidence of hemorrhages[7,31].

Comment

Why vacuum extraction procedures have a particularly high incidence of retinal hemorrhage in comparision to forceps operations is unclear. The majority of hemorrhages occur as a result of some type of spontaneous or induced obstetrical trauma but the precise mechanism is not yet established. Various etiologies have been suggested for retinal hemorrhages[71-74]. Most likely, retinal hemorrhage is in some fashion related to rapidly changing pressures within the fetal cranium during the birth process[71,72].

The hypothesis of Egge and co-workers[71] is that vacuum extraction causes temporary impairment of blood flow in the cavernous sinus and to the bridging veins which subsequently leads to venous stasis and resultant retinal bleeding. The apparent protective effect of outlet forceps may be to dampen pressure fluctuations within the fetal head by what Egge and co-workers[71] called a 'helmet' effect.

The clinical significance of retinal hemorrhage is unclear. Most data suggest that these lesions are transient events related to the birth process, with no permanent ill effects. The best information to date fails to find any correlation between such ocular findings at birth and later childhood visual development[7].

2.7 Nerve injury

Diagnosis

Nerve injuries are diagnosed by physical examination. An abducens (VI) palsy is diagnosed when failure of lateral eye abduction is noted during elicitation of the doll's-eyes reflex[75]. Involvement of the phrenic nerve accompanies a shoulder dystocia/brachial plexus injury and is manifested by respiratory embarrassment. Brachial plexus injuries result in characteristic motor paralysis of the affected limb. Other nerve injuries following vacuum extraction operations are rare (see Section 2.5 above).

Incidence

Nerve injuries, with the exception of brachial plexus injuries, are markedly uncommon[75-78]. Galbraith[75] reports discovering 24 transient abducens nerve palsies in 6886 infants (0.4%) admitted to a Level 1 neonatal service over a 10-year period. Vacuum extraction, midcavity forceps, and low forceps were identified as clinical associations in declining order of importance.

Comment

It is postulated that the abducens nerve is injured due to cranial distortion, which compresses the nerve during its transit through the petrous segment of the temporal bone[77,78]. There is an association between this injury and vacuum instrumental delivery, but data are scanty, the injury is rare and apparently transitory. Reliable estimates are not available for the incidence of the Weigert or phrenic nerve palsy but it is also clearly rare. Injuries to the brachial plexus are much more common, but still infrequent ($\leq 1/1000$ deliveries) and are described in detail above in Section 2.5[54,57,59,60].

IV.3 MATERNAL INJURIES

The most common maternal injury associated with vacuum extraction is episiotomy extension (Table IV.1)[79,80]. Close attention to detail during repair is mandatory. Particular care is necessary to diagnose occult fourth degree (rectal) extensions. Secondary breakdown of such lacerations/ extensions and formation of fistulae is uncommon and infection surprisingly infrequent. However, when such complications occur, the related problems are difficult for patient, family, and clinician. Rarely, maternal perineal injuries, including routine episiotomy, lead to serious complications such as necrotizing fasciitis[81–83].

Acute and chronic injury to the anal sphincter may accompany instrumental or spontaneous delivery with or without obvious laceration[84–86]. In some patients, these injuries result in long-term defecatory symptoms. It is unclear whether episiotomy protects from such dysfunction (or predisposes to it!). The long-term outcome of most such injuries remains unknown. Preliminary data suggest that vacuum extraction is *less* likely to result in chronic symptoms of rectal dysfunction than forceps delivery, although it is not clear why this might be so. Better controlled prospective studies with adequate control groups are needed.

Other maternal injuries are also possible. An extraction performed through an incompletely dilated cervix may result in a cervical laceration. If careful attention is not given to the cup margin when the ventouse is applied, redundant vaginal wall or cervix may be trapped under the edge and lacerated or crushed. Occasionally, if this injury occurs, frank blood is observed in the vacuum tubing or in the suction trap, alerting the clinician. *As with all instrumental deliveries, regardless of apparent ease, complete inspection of the birth canal after completing a vacuum-assisted delivery is mandatory.*

The basic prerequisites for repair of perineal injuries are simple: complete exposure, optimal positioning, strong illumination, and adequate analgesia/anesthesia. If evaluation proves difficult in the delivery suite, prompt transfer to an operating room for complete examination and repair is mandatory.

96

Birth canal lacerations are best repaired in layers using fine polyglycolic or polyglactin acid suture or, traditionally (but less desirably), with chromic suture material. Hematomas are evacuated as required, with hemostasis assured before the cavity is closed. Perineal lacerations involving the rectal sphincter and/or rectal mucosa are closed in layers with close attention to hemostasis and the re-approximation of normal anatomy. Good results are best assured by meticulous attention to detail, use of fine, non-strangulating suture, and close anatomic reconstruction. After surgery, patients should be fully apprised of such injuries and the possible implications if primary closure fails. Sitz baths may reduce patient distress postpartum and intermittent catheterization may be necessary. Analgesia is used as required. There is no evidence that the concurrent use of stool softeners, antibiotics or dietary supplements either aids healing or avoids the complications of infection or fistula formation.

Infections of vaginal lacerations or episiotomies are usually superficial and minor. However, if the perineal wound becomes infected, a common outcome is disruption with delayed healing by secondary intention. For superficial infections, treatment by simple wound exploration and debridement usually suffices. Antibiotics are administered if signs of cellulitis, induration or gross infection are present. Sitz baths and analgesics usually provide symptomatic relief.

On rare occasions, a birth-related infection can become severe or life-threatening[81–83]. While most of the serious cases of postpartum infection result from endometritis, other diagnoses are possible. Septic pelvic thrombophlebitis, pyelonephritis or necrotizing fasciitis are rare but potentially fatal infections demanding early diagnosis and aggressive management[79]. Readers are referred to standard obstetric textbooks for the management of these unusual complications.

REFERENCES

1. Radcliffe, W. (1989). *Milestones in Midwifery and the Secret Instrument*, p. 18. (San Francisco: Norman Publishing)
2. Speert, H. (1980). *Obstetrics and Gynecology in America, A History*, p. 118. (Baltimore: Waverly Press)
3. Lahat, E., Schiffer, J., Heyman, E., Dolphin, Z. and Starinski, R.I. (1987). Acute subdural hemorrhage: uncommon complication of vacuum extraction delivery. *Eur. J. Obstet. Gynaecol. Reprod. Biol.*, **25**, 255–8
4. Hanigan, W.C., Morgan, A.M., Stahlberg, L.K. and Hiller, J.L. (1990).

Tentorial hemorrhage associated with vacuum extraction. *Pediatr.*, **85**, 534–9

5. Hall, S.L. (1992). Simultaneous occurrence of intracranial and subgaleal hemorrhages complicating vacuum extraction delivery. *J. Perinatol.*, **12**, 185–7

6. Vacca, A. (1990). The place of the vacuum extractor in modern obstetric practice. *Fet. Med. Rev.*, **2**, 103–22

7. Vacca, A. (1992). *Handbook of Vacuum Extraction in Obstetric Practice.* (London: Edward Arnold)

8. Plauché, W.C. (1979). Fetal cranial injuries related to delivery with a Malmström vacuum extractor. *Obstet. Gynecol.*, **53**, 750–7

9. O'Grady, J.P. (1988). *Modern Instrumental Delivery.* (Baltimore: Williams & Wilkins)

10. Vacca, A. and Kierse, M.J.N.C. (1989). Instrumental vaginal delivery. In Chalmers, I., Eukin, M. and Keirse, M.J.N.C. (eds.) Effective Care in Pregnancy and Childbirth. (Oxford: Oxford University Press)

11. Florentino-Pineda, I., Ezuthachan, S.G., Sineni, L.G. and Kumar, S.P. (1994). Subgaleal hemorrhage in the newborn infant associated with silicone elastomer vacuum extractor. *J. Perinatol.*, **14**, 95–100

12. Laufe, L.E. and Berkus, M.D. (1992). Assisted Vaginal Delivery. (New York: McGraw-Hill Inc.)

13. Chenoy, R. and Johanson, R. (1992). A randomised prospective study comparing delivery with maternal silicone rubber vacuum extractor cups. *Br. J. Obstet. Gynaecol.*, **99**, 360–3

14. Thiery, M. (1985). Obstetric vacuum extraction. *Obstet. Gynecol. Annu.*, **14**, 73–111

15. Birenbaum, E., Robinson, G., Mashiach, S. and Brish, M. (1986). Skull subcutaneous emphysema – a rare complication of vacuum extraction and scalp electrodes. *Eur. J. Obstet. Gynecol. Reprod. Biol.*, **22**, 257–60

16. Volpe, J.J. (1987). *Neurology of the Newborn*, 2nd edn. (Philadelphia: WB Saunders Company)

17. Amosy, G. and Ahlander, K. (1960). Forceps delivery or vacuum extractor? A comparison over a five-year period. *Nord. Med.*, **64**, 839–42

18. Zilliacus, H. and Sjöstedt, E. (1961). In *Proceedings of the Third World Congress of the International Federation of Obstetrics and Gynecology*, Vienna, vol. 1, p. 84

19. Brandstrup, E. and Lange, P. (1961). Clinical experience with the vacuum extractor. In *Proceedings of the Third World Congress of the International Federation of Obstetrics and Gynecology*, pp. 207–11

20. Mishell, D. and Kelly, J.V. (1962). The obstetrical forceps and the vacuum extractor. An assessment of their compressive force. *Obstet. Gynecol.*, **19**, 204–6

21. Spritzer, T.D. (1962). Use of the vacuum extractor in obstetrics. *Am. J. Obstet. Gynecol.*, **83**, 307

22. Hammerstein, J. and Gromotke, R. (1962). The value of Malmström's extractor in operative obstetrics. *Obstet. Gynecol.*, **19**, 207–11

23. Guardino, A.N. and O'Brien, F.B. (1962). Preliminary experiences with Malmström's vacuum extractor. *Am. J. Obstet. Gynecol.*, **83**, 300–6

24. Munsat, T.L., Neerhout, R. and Nyirjesy, I. (1963). A comparative clinical study of the vacuum extractor and forceps. Part II. Evaluation of the newborn. *Am. J. Obstet. Gynecol.*, **85**, 1083–90

25. Roskowski, I., Borowski, R. and Kretowicz, J. (1963). Use of the vacuum extractor in fetal distress. *Am. J. Obstet. Gynecol.*, **87**, 253–7

26. Lasbrey, A.H., Orchard, C.D. and Crichton, D. (1964). A study of the relative merits and scope for vacuum extraction as opposed to forceps delivery. *S. Afr. J. Obstet. Gynaecol.*, **2**, 1–3

27. Malmström, T. (1964). The vacuum extractor. I. Indications and results. *Acta Obstet. Gynecol. Scand.*, **43**, 5–52

28. Barth, W.H. and Newton, M. (1965). The use of the vacuum extractor. *Am. J. Obstet. Gynecol.*, **91**, 403–6

29. Chalmers, J.A. (1965). The vacuum extractor in difficult delivery. *J. Obstet. Gynaecol. Br. Commonw.*, **72**, 889–91

30. St Vincent Buss, T. (1965). Vacuum extraction in the first stage of labor. *S. Afr. J. Obstet. Gynaecol.*, **3**, 53–7

31. Brat, T. (1965). Indications for and results of the use of the 'ventouse obstétricale' (a ten year study). *J. Obstet. Gynaecol. Br. Commonw.*, **72**, 883–8

32. Schenker, J.G. and Serr, D.M. (1967). Comparative study of delivery by vacuum extractor and forceps. *Am. J. Obstet. Gynecol.*, **98**, 32–9

33. Widen, J.A., Erez, S. and Steer, C.M. (1967). An evaluation of the vacuum extractor in a series of 201 cases. *Am. J. Obstet. Gynecol.*, **98**, 24–31

34. Broekhuizen, F.F., Washington, J.M., Johnson, F. and Hamilton, P.R. (1984). Vacuum extraction versus forceps delivery: indications and complications, 1979 to 1984. *Obstet. Gynecol.*, **57**, 571–7

35. Fahmy, K. (1971). Cephalhaematoma following vacuum extraction. *J. Obstet. Gynaecol. Br. Commonw.*, **78**, 369–72

36. Punnonen, R., Aro, P., Kuukankorpi, A. and Pustynen, P. (1986). Fetal and maternal effects of forceps and vacuum extraction. *Br. J. Obstet. Gynaecol.*, **93**, 1132–5

37. Ngan, H.Y.S., Tang, G.W.K. and Ma, H.K. (1986). Vacuum extractor: a safe instrument? *Aust. NZ J. Obstet. Gynaecol.*, **26**, 177–81

38. Wigglesworth, J.S. and Singer, D.B. (eds.) (1991). *Textbook of Fetal and Perinatal Pathology*. (Boston: Blackwell Scientific Publications)

39. Berkus, M.D., Ramamurthy, R.S., O'Connor, P.S. *et al.* (1985). Cohort study of silastic obstetric vacuum cup deliveries: I. Safety of the instrument. *Obstet. Gynecol.*, **66**, 503–9

40. Hernansanz, J., Munoz, F., Rodriguez, D., Soler, C. and Principe, C. (1984).

Subdural hematomas of the posterior fossa in normal weight newborns. *J. Neurosurg.*, **61**, 972–4

41. Romondov, A.P. and Brodsky, Y.S. (1987). Subdural hematomas in the newborn. *Surg. Neurol.*, **28**, 253–8

42. Holland, E. (1922). Cranial stress in the foetus during labour and on the effects of excessive stress on the intracranial contents: with an analysis of eighty-one cases of torn tentorium cerebelli and subdural cerebral hemorrhage. *J. Obstet. Gynaecol. Br. Emp.*, **29**, 551–71

43. Awon, M.P. (1973). The vacuum extractor – experimental demonstration of distortion of the foetal skull. *J. Perinat. Med.*, **1**, 291–2

44. Bjerre, I. and Dahlin, K. (1974). The longterm development of children delivered by vacuum extraction. *Dev. Med. Child Neurol.*, **16**, 378–81

45. Fenichel, G.M. (1993). *Clinical Pediatrics Neurology: A Sign and Symptoms Approach*, 2nd edn., pp. 99–103. (Philadelphia: WB Saunders Company)

46. Vanhaesebrouck, P.J., Poffyn, A., Camaert, J., De Baets, F., Van de Velde, E. and Thiery, M. (1990). Leptomeningeal cyst and vacuum extraction. *Acta Paediatr. Scand.*, **79**, 232–3

47. Hernandez, C. and Wendel, G.D. (1990). Shoulder dystocia. *Clin. Obstet. Gynecol.*, **33**, 526–34

48. Sandmire, H.F. and O'Halloin, T.J. (1988). Shoulder dystocia: its incidence and associated risk factors. *Int. J. Gynaecol. Obstet.*, **26**, 65–73

49. Gonik, B., Stringer, C.A. and Held, B. (1983). An alternate maneuver for management of shoulder dystocia. *Am. J. Obstet. Gynecol.*, **145**, 882–4

50. O'Leary, J.A. (1992). *Shoulder Dystocia and Birth Injury*. (New York: McGraw-Hill Inc.)

51. Resnik, R. (1980). Management of shoulder girdle dystocia. *Clin. Obstet. Gynecol.*, **23**, 559–64

52. Seigworth, G.R. (1966). Shoulder dystocia: review of 5 years experience. *Obstet. Gynecol.*, **28**, 764–7

53. Sandbury, E.C. (1985). The Zavanelli maneuver: a potentially revolutionary method for the resolution of shoulder dystocia. *Am. J. Obstet. Gynecol.*, **152**, 479–84

54. Acker, D.B., Sachs, B.P. and Friedman, E.A. (1985). Risk factors for shoulder dystocia. *Obstet. Gynecol.*, **66**, 762–8

55. Jennett, R.J., Tarby, T.J. and Kreinick, M.A. (1973). Brachial plexus palsy: an old problem revisited. *Am. J. Obstet. Gynecol.*, **117**, 51–6

56. Vassalos, E., Prevedourakis, C. and Paraschopoulou-Prevedouraki, P. (1968). Brachial plexus paralysis in the newborn. *Am. J. Obstet. Gynecol.*, **101**, 554–6

57. Tan, K.L. (1973). Brachial palsy. *J. Obstet. Gynaecol. Br. Commonw.*, **80**, 60–2

58. Gordon, M., Rich, H., Deutschberger, J. and Green, M. (1973). The immediate and longterm outcome of obstetric birth trauma. I. Brachial plexus paralysis. *Am. J. Obstet. Gynecol.*, **117**, 51–6

59. Specht, E.E. (1975). Brachial plexus palsy in the newborn. Incidence and prognosis. *Clin. Orthop. Relat. Res.*, **110**, 32–4

60. McFarland, L.V., Raskin, M., Daling, F.R. and Benedetti, T.J. (1986). Erbs/Duchenne's palsy: a consequence of fetal macrosomia and method of delivery. *Obstet. Gynecol.*, **68**, 784–8

61. Benedetti, T.J. and Gabbe, S.G. (1978). Shoulder dystocia. A complication of fetal macrosomia and prolonged second stage of labor with midpelvic delivery. *Obstet. Gynecol.*, **52**, 526–9

62. Gilbert, A. and Whitaker, I. (1991). Obstetric brachial plexus lesions. *(Br.) J. Hand Surg.*, **16**, 489–91

63. Graham, J.M., Blanco, J.D. and Wen, T. (1992). The Zavanelli Maneuver: a different perspective. *Obstet. Gynecol.*, **79**, 883–4

64. O'Leary, J.A. and Cuva, A. (1992). Abdominal rescue after failed cephalic replacement. *Obstet. Gynecol.*, **80**, 514–16

65. O'Leary, J.A. and Leonetti, H. (1990). Shoulder dystocia, prevention and treatment. *Am. J. Obstet. Gynecol.*, **162**, 5–9

66. American College of Obstetricians and Gynecologists (1994). *Operative Vaginal Delivery.* Technical Bulletin No. 196. (Washington DC: American College of Obstetricians and Gynecologists)

67. Van Roosmalen, J. (1991). Symphyseotomy – a re-appraisal for the developing world. In Studd, J. (ed.) *Progress in Obstetrics and Gynaecology*, vol. 9, pp. 149–62. (Edinburgh: Churchill-Livingstone)

68. Gebbie, D. (1982). Symphysiotomy. *Clin. Obstet. Gynecol.*, **9**, 663–83

69. Shute, W.B. (1962). Management of shoulder dystocia with the Shute parallel forceps. *Am. J. Obstet. Gynecol.*, **84**, 936–9

70. Kuit, J.A., Eppinga, H.G., Wallenburg, H.C. and Huikeshoven, F.J. (1993). A randomized comparison of vacuum extraction delivery with a rigid and a pliable cup. *Obstet. Gynecol.*, **82**, 280–84

71. Egge, K., Lyng, G. and Maltau, J.M. (1981). Effect of instrumental delivery on the frequency and severity of retinal hemorrhages in the newborn. *Acta Obstet. Gynecol. Scand.*, **60**, 153–5

72. Ehlers, N., Jensen, F.K. and Hansen, K.B. (1974). Retinal hemorrhages in the newborn. Comparison of delivery by forceps and by vacuum extraction. *Acta Ophthalmol.*, **52**, 73–82

73. Giles, C.L. (1960). Retinal hemorrhages in the newborn. *Am. J. Opthalmol.*, **49**, 1005–11

74. Painter, M.J. and Bergman, I. (1982). Obstetrical trauma to the neonatal central and peripheral nervous system. *Semin. Perinatol.*, **6**, 89–104

75. Galbraith, R.S. (1994). Incidence of neonatal sixth nerve palsy in relation to mode of delivery. *Am. J. Obstet. Gynecol.*, **170**, 1158–9

76. Levine, M.G., Holyrode, J., Woods, J.R., Jr., Siddigi, T.A., Scott, M. and Miodounik, M. (1984). Birth trauma: incidence and predisposing factors. *Obstet. Gynecol.*, **63**, 792–5

77. Reisner, S.H., Perlman, M., Ben-Tovim, N. and Dubrawski, C. (1971). Transient lateral rectus muscle paresis in the newborn infant. *J. Pediatr.*, **78**, 461–5

78. deGrauw, A.J., Rottenveel, J. and Cruysberg, J.R. (1983). Transient sixth nerve paralysis in the newborn infant. *Neuropaediatrics*, **14**, 164–5

79. Sleep, J., Roberts, J. and Chalmers, I. (1989). Care during the second stage of labour. In Chalmers, I., Eukin, M. and Keirse, M. (eds.) *Effective Care in Pregnancy and Childbirth*, pp. 1129–99. (Oxford: Oxford University Press)

80. Sweet, R.L. and Gibbs, R.S. (1990). Postpartum infection. In Sweet, R.L. and Gibbs, R.S. (eds.) *Infectious Diseases of the Female Genital Tract*, 2nd edn., pp. 356–82. (Baltimore: Williams & Wilkins)

81. Sky, K.K. and Eschenbach, D.A. (1979). Fatal perineal cellulitis from an episiotomy site. *Obstet. Gynecol.*, **54**, 292–8

82. Dellinger, E.P. (1981). Severe necrotizing soft tissue infections. *J. Am. Med. Assoc.*, **246**, 1717–21

83. Sultan, A.H., Kamm, M.A., Bartram, C.I. and Hudson, C.N. (1993). Anal sphincter trauma during instrumental delivery. *Int. J. Gynaecol. Obstet.*, **43**, 263–70

84. Combs, C.A., Robertson, P.A., Laros, R.K. Jr (1990). Risk factors for third-degree perineal lacerations in forceps and vacuum deliveries. *Am. J. Obstet. Gynecol.*, **163**, 100–4

85. Sultan, A.H., Kamm, M.A., Bartram, C.I. *et al.* (1992). Third degree tears: incidence, risk factors, and poor clinical outcome after primary sphincter repair. *Br. Med. J.*, **308**, 887–91

86. Pape, W.E. and Wigglesworth, J.S. (1979). *Haemorrhage, Ischaemia and the Perinatal Brain*. (Philadelphia: JB Lippincott)

V

Legal issues

For every man shall bear his own burden . . . for whatsoever a man soweth, that shall he also reap.

The Epistle of Paul the Apostle
Galatians 6:5–7[1]

Without question, allegations of medical negligence and medical malpractice have influenced modern obstetric practice. While the importance of this influence is controversial, its presence is not. Modern clinicians understand the importance of being well informed and knowledgeable concerning these matters. The following section contains an introduction to the legal principles and aspects of medical-legal analysis which are relevant to obstetric vacuum extraction procedures.

V.1 THE PROCESS AND NATURE OF MEDICOLEGAL ANALYSIS

State laws governing medical negligence within the United States are not uniform. However, there are common elements. To establish a case of medical negligence/medical malpractice the injured party must prove that the accused physician:

(a) Owed a duty of care to the patient;

(b) Failed by act or omission to provide the appropriate level of ordinary care required (i.e., failed to meet the requisite standard of care); and

(c) That such failure was the cause in fact (or, proximate cause) of the injury.

1.1 Basic analytic inquiries

While legal analysis in a potential medical malpractice case may ultimately prove complex, at its inception, the approach is rather straight-forward. All potential medical negligence cases begin with an injury. This injury must have some temporal or causal relationship to the medical/surgical care under investigation.

The cost of investigating and pursuing medical negligence litigation is exceedingly high in comparison to most other types of personal injury law suits. Therefore, as a practical matter, the injury in a medical malpractice proceeding must be permanent, disabling, or disfiguring to warrant the serious attention of a lawyer. Transient or trivial injuries are rarely the subject matter of malpractice litigation. The Latin adage expresses this well – *de minimis non curat lex* (the law does not concern itself with trifles).

Once the seriousness of the injury has been confirmed, primary legal analysis attempts to answer the following basic questions:

(1) Did medical science at the time of the occurrence have the means to prevent the injury which occurred?

(2) Is it more likely than not that the accused physician failed, by act or omission, to meet the required standard of care?

(3) It is more likely than not that the injury was the result of the physician's failure, by act or omission, to meet the required standard of care?

1.2 Standard of care

In a medical negligence case the standard of care is not a fixed formula. Rather, it is a dynamic process which changes over time to accommodate new technologies and the accumulated knowledge and experience of medical practitioners. Knowledge, skill, care, and diligence are the defining elements in establishing standards for medical and/or surgical care. Significant deficiencies in any one of these elements or a combination of them may result in allegations of substandard care or 'negligence'[2]. The additional element of 'under the same or similar circumstances' is either stated or implied in order to address the diverse conditions under which a physician may be required to render treatment. This provision allows that under some circumstances the physician may be justified in providing a lesser measure or quality of medical care than that which is required under optimal conditions. This could occur because of limitations imposed by the severity of the patient's condition, critical time constraints, or the unavailability of staff or technical support. Whether or not a physician is justified in initiating care or treatment knowing such limitations exist, depends upon the reasonableness of his/her actions at the time in question. Such issues can only be properly evaluated by close attention to the unique facts of a specific case.

While the precise words used to define the requisite standard of care vary from jurisdiction to jurisdiction, there is a fundamental similarity concerning what is legally required. The standard of care does not demand practice at a level of excellence or even above average performance. It requires only 'average' or 'ordinary' practice. Applying this standard, in grade school terms, the physician is only negligent when his or her performance is 'C minus' or lower when compared with other physicians in the same field of specialization.

The question of whether or not a physician fell below acceptable standards of practice is largely determined following a review of the facts of the case by a well-qualified physician with broad-based experience in performing the same procedures who is able to assess the particular circumstances confronting the accused. This is the role of the expert witness.

Most jurisdictions require that the expert witnesses be a practicing physician in the same field of specialization as the physician whose conduct is under investigation. While some jurisdictions do permit medical experts to testify concerning the standard of care required of physicians practicing in another medical specialty (other than their own), it is, at the very least required that these experts demonstrate knowledge of the applicable standard.

Ordinarily, no single document or pronouncement constitutes a definitive statement of the applicable standard of care. Not surprisingly, both medical literature and statements by learned bodies play an important role in establishing medical standards but are by no means the only source. The sources of information which are often relied upon in determining the requisite standard of care may include but are not limited to the following:

(1) Information generated by *legitimate* scientific and medical investigations;

(2) Experience and knowledge acquired through medical school, internship, residency, fellowship program, postgraduate study, and the actual practice of medicine;

(3) Information documented within standard medical textbooks.

(4) Information documented within referred medical journals;

(5) Information communicated by medical and scientific investigators and recognized medical authorities at educational seminars and training sessions;

(6) Data obtained through communication with professional colleagues concerning their experience or training;

(7) Standards, policies, procedures, protocols, and recommendations promulgated by the hospital or department of obstetrics and gynecology where the physician practices;

(8) Policies, procedures, protocols and recommendations approved and formulated by professional organizations, medical societies, or other learned bodies;

(9) The recommendations and precautions reported by manufacturers of medical instruments and pharmacologic products; and

(10) Statutory enactments and the findings, or recommendations of government agencies or organizations.

Despite these multiple components, there is almost always a clearly defined consensus within the medical community as to what is and is not appropriate medical care It is rare that a knowledgeable physician can honestly say that he does not know what the standard of care requires within his own field of specialization[2].

V.2 OBSTETRIC INJURIES THAT ARE COMMONLY THE SUBJECT OF LAWSUITS: VACUUM EXTRACTION DELIVERY

Injuries associated with instrumental delivery procedures, which most often trigger medical/legal investigation include trauma to both the mother and her infant. The major categories include:

2.1 Fetal injuries

(a) Hypoxic brain injury.

(b)   Adverse neurologic effects (short term and potential long term).

(c)   Cerebral contusion and intracranial hemorrhages.

(d)   Shoulder dystocia/brachial plexus injury.

(e)   Injuries to the spinal cord or cervical spine.

(f)   Nerve injuries.

(g)   Local scalp injury: laceration, abrasion, ecchymosis, or necrosis, especially accompanied by infection or symptomatic anemia.

(h)   Serious scalp injury such as subgaleal (subaponeurotic) hemorrhage, or large cephalhematoma with or without underlying skull fracture.

(i)   Eye injury or blindness.

(j)   Fractures (clavicle, humerus, femur, skull).

(k)   Death.

2.2   Maternal injuries

(a)   Vaginal lacerations.

(b)   Uterine rupture or cervical laceration.

(c)   Episiotomy extensions into sphincter or rectum.

(d)   Bladder and urethral injury.

(e)   Fistula formation (bladder and bowel).

(f)   Severe hemorrhage and/or infection.

(g)   Death.

The above-listed maternal injuries are most commonly associated with forceps procedures involving either forcible rotation or traction. However, many of these injuries have occurred (albeit with far less frequency and ordinarily lesser trauma) in vacuum extraction procedures. This may happen where the operator has failed to remove redundant maternal tissue from beneath the vacuum cup before exerting traction or where excessive force, incorrectly oriented force, or an unusual number of traction efforts were attempted.

While it is exceedingly difficult to identify conduct which is presumptively malpractice or negligence *per se*, one can be reasonably confident that an obvious violation of well established requirements and conditions for safe instrumental delivery, which are orthodoxy in modern

American obstetric practice, will almost certainly be considered substandard practice. The basic conditions or requirements for safe instrumental delivery are discussed in the current ACOG Bulletins concerning instrumental delivery and in well established obstetric literature on the subject[3-8]. The basic requirements include:

(1) Clear medical indications for the procedure;

(2) Absence of cephalopelvic disproportion;

(3) Concomitant preparation for Cesarean delivery with immediate availability of all requisite personnel in the case of a trial of instrumental delivery;

(4) Undertaking all cases of instrumentation as if they were truly a trial, with the requirement that the obstetrician remain willing to abandon an attempted instrumental delivery in favor of a Cesarean operation when no descent occurs following reasonable traction effort(s); and

(5) An operator/surgeon with demonstrable knowledge and skill in performing deliveries with the chosen instrument (either vacuum extractor or forceps).

It must be understood that mere compliance with these conditions neither justifies a specific instrumental delivery operation nor affirms that the obstetrician has met the acceptable standards of practice.

Midpelvic forceps rotation is particularly condemned by many knowledgeable investigators on the grounds that it is likely to cause severe lacerations and trauma to maternal tissues when performed by operators lacking sufficient experience, skill, or caution. There is a general consensus among medical authors that midpelvic extractions, performed with the vacuum extractor have a lower incidence of maternal trauma than forceps operations from the same station. In some studies the incidence of significant maternal trauma was so low as to be accounted all but negligible by the investigator. Therefore, from the standpoint of potential litigation, the burden of persuasion will be upon the accused physician to justify performing a midforceps rotational procedure as opposed to the more benign alternative of a vacuum extraction operation or a manual rotation.

V.3   SOURCES OF ERROR AND CRITICISM: VACUUM EXTRACTION PROCEDURES

A reasonably sophisticated awareness of what criterion are used to assess physician conduct can be derived from a review of court files, insurance company reports, medical case reviews and the commentary of seasoned litigators and medical experts. These sources indicated that the bulk of malpractice litigation involving instrumental delivery derives from four broad categories of obstetric errors:

(1) Failure to exercise adequate and informed medical judgment when assessing what cases are appropriate for an instrumental operation and when that intervention should take place.

(2) Failure to understand or accept the limitations of the procedure itself and plan in advance for possible failures.

(3) Failure to timely abandon a trial of instrumental delivery. Particularly the failure to eschew improperly prolonged, repeated or excessive traction efforts in the presence of poor (or no) progress.

(4) Failure to properly assess the position of the fetal head in relationship to the pelvic outlet and the attempting to advance the fetal head by traction against the resistance of an unfavorable pelvic diameter or fetal position (i.e., unrecognized cephalopelvic disproportion).

3.1 Potential legal allegations and defenses

A more concrete and practical insight into the nature of medical-legal criticism of physicians performing vacuum extraction procedures can be obtained by examining the allegations and defenses raised in actual cases filed with the courts. The following litanies of potential legal allegations and defenses are by no means exhaustive. Their purpose is to identify common patterns of medical-legal claims, accusations, and defenses.

Allegations

(1) *Failure to properly assess the delivery as one that could be safely accomplished by a vaginal instrumental procedure.*

    (a) Absence of an appropriate indication for instrumental delivery.

    (b) Proceeding when the cervix is not completely dilated, or the head is not engaged.

    (c) Improper use of the vacuum extractor to deliver a premature infant, resulting in intracranial hemorrhage, or permanent neurologic injury.

(d) Improper use of the vacuum extractor in the presence of fetal malpositioning (face, brow, etc.) resulting in intracranial or serious soft tissue injury.

(2) Improper use of vacuum extraction in the presence of known or suspected *cephalopelvic or fetopelvic disproportion* when the physician knew or should have known that delivery could not be safely accomplished vaginally.

(3) *Failure to alert the pediatrician and responsible nursing staff* concerning the need to monitor a newborn for signs of intracranial hemorrhage in a complicated case when the obstetrician knew or should have known that the use of vacuum extraction equipment could cause this potentially lethal and injurious complication.

(4) *Failure to prepare in advance for immediate Cesarean delivery in a trial of instrumented vaginal delivery* knowing that the procedure could prove unsuccessful and the potential delay injurious to the unborn infant.

(5) *Improperly undertaking a trial of vacuum extraction in a facility/hospital which does not have the capability of accomplishing an emergency Cesarean delivery,* resulting in severe hypoxic brain injury or death to the infant.

(6) *Failure of the operating surgeon or his support staff to insure that all operating room personnel required for an emergency Cesarean delivery* (including but not limited to anesthesia) *are actually present* (or immediately available) *before undertaking a trial of vacuum extraction* with resulting delay in accomplishing an emergency Cesarean delivery and brain injury or death to the infant.

(7) Failure to promptly perform a Cesarean delivery:

(a) After the onset of fetal distress when the physician knew or should have known that further trials of vacuum extraction could not assure a safe and prompt delivery.

(b) Following a failed vacuum extraction, in the presence of fetal distress or presumed cephalopelvic or fetopelvic disproportion.

(8) Failure to use the vacuum extraction equipment with that level of skill, knowledge and training ordinarily exercised by obstetricians under the same or similar circumstances:

(a) Improperly attempting an active rotation of the fetal head by rotation of the extractor cup resulting in laceration or other injury to the fetal scalp.

    (b) Failure to remove redundant maternal tissue from beneath the extractor cup resulting in maternal injury, including:

        (i)   Injury to maternal urinary tract or bowel.

        (ii) Significant hemorrhage and/or infection.

        (iii) Laceration and scarring of the birth canal.

        (iv) Fistula formation.

(9) Application of excessive vacuum force, excessively prolonged vacuum force, or excessive traction (multiple applications of traction and/or multiple cup detachments) in the presence of obvious resistance and presumed cephalopelvic disproportion resulting in fetocranial fracture and/or obvious disruption of intracranial vascular structures.

(10) Failure to properly manage fetopelvic dystocia (i.e. shoulder girdle dystocia) following a vacuum assisted delivery by controlled and directed traction force with resulting nerve injury resulting in either an Erb/Duchenne, Klumpke, or Weigart paralysis or other infant injuries, including death. This could include:

    (a) Improper and/or excessive traction force applied to the cervical spine.

    (b) Improperly failing to consider the possibility of shoulder dystocia as suggested by a review of the mother's prior obstetric history, prenatal course, ultrasonic data, or course in labor.

    (c) Failing to properly evaluate fetal size or failing to make necessary preparations for appropriate anesthesia and assistance prior to an attempt at vacuum delivery.

    (d) Improperly failing to timely diagnose and appropriately manage shoulder dystocia through the use of standard obstetric maneuvers (McRoberts', Wood's cork-screw, etc.) with resulting maternal or fetal injuries.

(11) Failure to maintain diligent surveillance of fetal heart tones, an electronic fetal heart rate tracing, or other indicators of fetal well being throughout the course of the instrumental trial/delivery with resulting brain injury or death. This could include:

    (a) Failure to timely detect cord prolapse/compromise occasioned

111

by impingement, traction or descent against the cord during a trial of instrumental delivery resulting in brain injury or death.

(12) Failure to properly inform mother and family of the nature, purposes, risks and alternatives to the procedure actually performed.

(13) Failure to provide for the proper supervision of an inexperienced or inadequately trained physician practitioner (or resident physician in training) by a well-qualified and fully trained staff obstetrician.

Telephone supervision of junior or inexperienced personnel during an instrumental delivery is rarely defensible as an adequate method of assuring the safety and well being of either the mother or her unborn infant. Likewise, supervision of one resident by another more senior resident is particularly vulnerable to criticism, depending upon the technical demands/complexity of the delivery undertaken. Ordinarily, most senior residents have performed few difficult extractions and are thus poorly qualified as instructors for such technically demanding operations. It should be understood that the inexperienced or inadequately trained physician has an independent responsibility to consult with and obtain the direct supervision of a fully trained practitioner, experienced in vacuum delivery procedures, before attempting a complicated procedure. This applies whenever the inexperienced physician either knows or should know that the procedure is beyond his/her skill or competency.

In the legal arena the physician accused can dispute the allegations of wrong doing by offering counter-proofs which demonstrate that he or she acted in a reasonably prudent, and legally defensible manner which was consistent with sound medical practice and conformed to the requisite standard of care. Common patterns of defense raised in response to allegations of negligent instrumental delivery include the following:

Defenses

(1) Offering affirmative proof which defines the standard of care for the case in a manner which exculpates the accused physician or hospital employee.

(2) Disputing the definition of the standard of care relied upon by the plaintiff's expert. This might include:

(a) Offering proof that the medical principles or reasoning relied upon by the opposing expert's opinion are unsound and/or unsupported by established medical/scientific teachings.

(b) Offering proof of an alternative version of the facts which exculpates the physician defendant.

(3) Offering proof of alternative causes for the birth injuries, i.e. that the actual mechanism or cause was not within the control of the accused physician or that it was not the physician's responsibility to prevent the occurence.

(4) Denying that the injured party is able to prove, by the greater weight of medical and scientific evidence, that any negligent act or omission of the accused physician or medical practitioner(s) caused the injury.

(5) Offering proof that the accused obstetrician reasonably relied upon nursing staff and house physicians to monitor the fetal and maternal well being and timely report any significant changes in their status.

(6) Offering proof that but for the negligent failure of nursing staff or hospital physicians to timely report significant changes in maternal or fetal well being, the accused obstetrician would have provided timely and appropriate medical/surgical intervention.

(7) Admitting that there was negligent conduct which caused the injury complained of, while denying that the plaintiff (injured party) is entitled to the amount of money damages requested (i.e. simply arguing for a lesser monetary damage award).

(8) Offering proof that the injury suffered by the patient is a known risk or complication of the procedure performed which can occur even with the exercise of ordinary knowledge, skill, care and diligence on the part of the physician and his or her support staff.

This defense should be linked with affirmative proof of informed consent. The defense must either establish the patient's knowledge and actual acceptance of the risk involved or offer proof that a reasonable person, similarly situated, would have accepted this same risk.

(9) Offering proof that the patients own negligent conduct caused or contributed to cause the injury.

Charging the patient with negligent conduct can be a problematic defense. This approach has limited appeal unless there is clear proof of patient misconduct which makes her unappealing or unsympathetic to the jury. Such charges might include evidence that the patient failed to make herself available for follow-up care or examination, failed to timely alert the physician to significant changes in her condition, did not comply with the doctor's instructions, and/or failed to abstain from using harmful or addictive substances such as alcohol or various drugs.

V.4 DOCUMENTATION

4.1 The procedure note

Detailed and complete documentation of all relevant clinical information concerning a vacuum extraction delivery is mandatory. As discussed in Chapter II, Instruments, indications, and issues, Section 3.1, this documentation should take the form of operative dictation and should include, but is not limited to:

(1)   Indication(s) for the procedure;

(2)   Anesthesia;

(3)   Personnel present;

(4)   Instrument(s) used;

(5)   Station, position and defection of the fetal head at commencement of the operation; and

(6)   Complications and a detailed description of how they were managed.

4.2 The medical record

When a case comes under legal review, close examination and investigation of the medical record must be anticipated. The plaintiff's lawyer will search out internal and logical inconsistencies between the events described in the operative report and the observations documented by physicians or nurses in attendance. Both the lawyer and his consulting expert will be quick to note any obvious failure of the operative report to logically explain or reasonably justify the injury inflicted.

An erroneous but surprisingly popular belief is that an obstetrician who says little or nothing within the operative note or case dictation will later, with the assistance of his lawyer and perhaps a consulting obstetrical expert, be better able to formulate a well thought out 'statement of the facts' which is persuasive and exculpatory. The underlying assumption is that if limited specific information is reported in the medical record, there is greater latitude in persuasively 'explaining away' subsequent charges of medical negligence. Such vague, general or formulaic operative reports or case dictations are easily identified and are highly vulnerable to criticism. Such reports are immediately suspect and usually heighten rather than diminish an attorney's willingness to investigate and pursue litigation.

Physicians should also be alerted to the hazards of going to the other extreme. Executing an excessively complex, obsessively detailed medical record, or providing an exhaustive litany of causes which could possibly account for a birth injury, is discouraged. The suggestion of causes which are rare, remote or speculative usually only assures that the physician will later be made to appear either suspiciously defensive or simply ridiculous.

To be accurate, reliable, and credible the case dictation should be prepared at or near the time of the events. The purpose of clear, precise, and detailed documentation is to demonstrate that the obstetrician was aware of all relevant clinical information and thereafter proceeded in a reasonable, rational, and logical manner consistent with well-established medical and obstetrical principles. Precise and accurate recording of times, at critical junctures, goes a long way toward proving that the physician acted reasonably and with due diligence in the face of fetal distress or similar urgent clinical circumstances. The operative report and other medical record notations which are prepared must be consistent with 'good medical practice'. That is, the record should contain accurate information in sufficient detail to document the care provided and to assure effective communication for continuation of care by subsequent treating physicians. This document, assuming it accurately reflects the actual events that transpired, is of great value in defending against subsequent allegations of medical negligence.

V.5   COMMUNICATION

Failed communication is the most significant factor motivating the injured patient to seek out a malpractice lawyer. The ability to speak to patients in a manner which assures understanding is the best means of avoiding antagonism, fear or anger on the part of those who have suffered injury or loss. Lawyers interviewing prospective clients are often privy to the anger, outrage, and alienation which inevitably follow the patient's loss of trust and confidence in his/her doctor. It is the wound of betrayal, not avarice, which first sets a lawsuit in motion. Common complaints voiced by malpractice litigants to lawyers include: 'I told him something was wrong but he said it was nothing . . . well it *was* something', 'she ignored what I told her', 'she talked to me in technical jargon I couldn't understand', 'after I was hurt (my baby was hurt) she never really explained what had happened, she just stopped talking'. Many times these litigants describe the behavior of their physicians as abrupt, arrogant, distant, unfeeling, inconsiderate, and even abusive.

5.1 Talking to patients

The critical junctures, out of which failed or ineffective communication most often gives rise to malpractice litigation in instrumental delivery, include:

(1) When the physician informs the patient that her infant (or she) has suffered serious injury; and

(2) When the physician discusses the nature, purpose, risks, and alternatives to a recommended surgical procedure as part of a consent.

Clear and effective communication requires a precise and exacting vocabulary, a common understanding of the meaning of the words used, and ongoing observations which confirm the accurate transmission of thought and shared understanding. It is the obligation of the physician to not only speak precisely but also to confirm that the patient has understood. The latter is best measured by asking the patient to paraphrase what the physician has said and by encouraging questions. Through effective communication the physician can reveal his or her genuine interest, compassionate concern, and respect.

5.2 Communicating adverse outcomes

Timing is critical in communicating an adverse outcome. It is imperative that the patient and family be informed, whenever possible, of difficulties as they are encountered, the efforts being employed to overcome those difficulties, and the adverse outcome which the physician and his staff are attempting to avoid. It is a capital mistake to misinform the family that 'all is well' despite a developing problem and then suddenly do an 'about face' and communicate the fact that a death or a serious injury has occurred. When bad news is unanticipated and thrust upon a patient unexpectedly, the response is often one of anger, disbelief, and distrust.

When an injury has occurred, the physician must be sensitive to the needs of his patient and carefully assess her ability to hear and discuss without being overwhelmed by strong emotion. The physician's approach should not be motivated by his own anxieties or fears; arriving with a phalanx of hospital officials and approaching the patient with diplomatic formality is ill-advised. Rather, this should be a private moment of shared grief and loss as a natural outgrowth of the compassionate concern and trust which has been patiently cultivated throughout the relationship. If the foundation of this relationship has been built in an honest and sincere fashion it will withstand remarkable stresses.

The physician's communications should be candid, direct, and caring. When the circumstances leading to death or injury are known, they should be shared. If the causes of injury are not fully known or understood, the physician should frankly admit that he/she does not know and explain why. These discussions are difficult for all involved and time consuming. This shared experience of loss and grief mark the beginning of healing for both patient and physician; it should never be avoided or given short shrift.

V.6   CONSENT

The importance of 'informed consent' as a basis for malpractice litigation is overstated. Anxious physicians mistakenly believe that obtaining an airtight informed consent from their patients provides a foolproof defense against malpractice suits. In fact, allegations that a physician failed to properly obtain an informed patient consent rarely stand alone as the basis for malpractice litigation. Allegations of a negligent act or omission in treatment almost invariably make up the core of a plaintiff's case. The allegation of failure to obtain an informed consent functions as a 'harmonic chord', allowing the plaintiff to offer testimony that the physician lacked respect, candor, compassion or humanity, and thus is likely to be guilty of the substantive act or omission which is really the plaintiff's chief allegation.

A physician, in obtaining a patient's consent to treatment or surgery, must discuss the nature, purpose, risks, and alternatives to the procedure in a manner consistent with what other physicians in the same field of specialization would do under the same or similar circumstances. The physician is required to advise his patients of those risks which a reasonable person would consider material to deciding whether or not to undergo the recommended procedure. To prove that an injury occurred as a direct result of the physician's failure to properly obtain an informed consent, the plaintiff must prove that she would not have accepted the risks or undergone the procedure had the true facts been known. In most jurisdictions, she must also persuade the jury that a 'reasonable person' in her same circumstances would not have accepted the risk.

A common myth among physicians is that remote or rare risks need not be communicated. Whether or not a risk is remote or even rare does not alone determine whether it should be discussed. The physician must engage in a reasoned risk vs. benefit analysis. If the benefit is small and the risk is remote but catastrophic (death, paralysis, blindness, deformity, etc.) it is prudent to inform the patient of the risk and its likelihood of occurrence. On the other hand, if the benefit is great (life-saving intervention) and the risk is remote and transient or trivial in nature, it is unnecessary to disclose that information. Obviously, this risk/benefit analysis varies from situation to situation and must be tailored to the particular patient whenever possible.

Fundamental to the process of consent is active participation by the patient in decision-making and her acceptance of responsibility for informed choices. It is of little value psychologically to have negotiated the technical requirements of effectively disclosing the required information only to permit the patient to surrender the choice entirely to the physician. The physician should insist that his patient accept some responsibility for choosing between available alternatives.

REFERENCES

1. The Holy Bible. Authorized King James Version, p. 1194. (1947) (Chicago: Spencer Press)
2. O'Grady, J.P. and McIlhargie, C.J. (1995). Instrumental delivery. In O'Grady,

J.P., Gimovsky, M.L. and McIlhargie, C.J. (eds.) *Operative Obstetrics.* (Baltimore: Williams & Wilkins)

3. O'Grady, J.P. (1988). *Modern Instrumental Delivery.* (Baltimore: Williams & Wilkins)

4. Laufe, L.E. and Berkus, M.D. (1992). *Assisted Vaginal Delivery: Obstetrical Forceps and Vacuum Extraction Techniques.* (New York: McGraw-Hill)

5. Dennen, P.C. (1990). *Dennen's Forceps Deliveries,* 3rd edn. (Philadelphia: FA Davis)

6. American College of Obstetrics and Gynecology (1994). *Operative Vaginal Delivery. Technical Bulletin #196.* (Washington D.C.: American College of Obstetrics and Gynecology)

7. American College of Obstetrics and Gynecology (1991). *Operative Vaginal Delivery. Technical Bulletin #152.* (Washington D.C.: American College of Obstetrics and Gynecology)

8. American College of Obstetrics and Gynecology (1989). *Obstetric Forceps. ACOG Committee Opinion #71.* (Washington D.C.: American College of Obstetrics and Gynecology)

VI

RISK ASSESSMENT

> *There is a time to let things happen and a time to make things happen.*
>
> Hugh Prather

VI.1 OVERVIEW

Injuries to the mother, her infant or both are possible during instrumental Cesarean or spontaneous delivery.[...] When modern obstetric management is considered, in fact, trauma occurs largely in premature infants (< 1500 g) following difficult deliveries or in association with malpositioning or malpresentations. In instrumental deliveries, injuries result from unanticipated shoulder dystocia, difficult or inaccurate instrument applications, inadequate analgesia/anesthesia, poor technique, failure to recognize malpresentation or subtle degrees of fetopelvic disproportion, or supply from bad luck. Cesarean delivery does not preclude fetal injury. This is particularly true in instances of malpresentation or for premature infants in the setting of fetal distress. The manipulations necessary to extract these fetuses can result in injuries similar to those seen following vaginal extractions, although the level of risk is lower. Fortunately, most delivery injuries are neither severe nor life-threatening. While the vast majority of harm resulting from

VI

Risk assessment

It is not to those who devise imperfect substitutes for valuable instruments, or temporary palliatives for important operations, in order that the awkward and ignorant may imperfectly perform what the skillful and instructed only should attempt, or are capable of accomplishing, that is (where) praise is to be awarded.

Issac Hayes
Elements of Physics, 1831[1]

There is a time to let things happen and a time to make things happen

Hugh Prather[2]

VI.1 OVERVIEW

Injuries to the mother, her infant or both are possible during instrumental, Cesarean or spontaneous delivery[3–8]. When modern obstetric management is considered, *in toto*, trauma occurs largely in premature infants (< 1500 g) following difficult deliveries or in association with malpositioning or malpresentations. In instrumental deliveries, injuries result from unanticipated shoulder dystocia, difficult or inaccurate instrument applications, inadequate analgesia/anesthesia, poor technique, failure to recognize malpresentation or subtle degrees of fetopelvic disproportion, or simply from bad luck. Cesarean delivery does not preclude fetal injury. This is particularly true in instances of malpresentation or for premature infants in the setting of fetal distress. The manipulations necessary to extract these fetuses can result in injuries similar to those seen following vaginal extractions, although the level of risk is lower. Fortunately, most delivery injuries are neither severe nor life-threatening. While the vast majority of harm resulting from

121

instrumental delivery is of trivial consequence, serious and even fatal injuries are possible (see Chapter IV, Complications and birth injuries).

While there is extensive clinical experience with instrumental delivery[6,8–12], there are unresolved concerns about the long-term effects of vaginal operative delivery procedures[13–20]. Nonetheless, the data from several large follow-up studies are reassuring, indicating few, if any, long-term adverse effects[16,17,19,20]. However, there are several problems with such studies. Inevitably, in such investigations, cases are lost to follow-up, such as procedure-related deaths. In addition, adequate controls are not always available and in the various reports the period of follow-up and methods of determining outcome are variable.

Accepting these limitations, the available data may be fairly interpreted to indicate that permanent neurological sequelae from assisted delivery are rare unless substantial trauma occurs in association with prematurity and/or birth asphyxia[10,16,17,19,20–21]. As with most obstetric untoward events, *pregnancy antecedents rather than delivery events are most important in predicting long-term neonatal outcome*[22]. This is not to suggest that injury cannot or does not occur with an individual birth. It is only a reminder that the *major* risks for long-term neurological dysfunction are genetic or developmental factors[23–25].

The critical variables which determine the safety and appropriateness of an instrumental delivery include the difficulty of the contemplated procedure, the skill of the operator, and the fetal condition at the time the procedure is performed. There is minimal debate concerning fetal risk from simple outlet procedures, regardless of the instrument chosen. These operations are generally recognized as safe[8,26]. However, even such simple operations are associated with an increased incidence of potentially complex maternal perineal trauma largely related to episiotomy and its inherent complications[3].

Most concern for fetal safety arises from mid-cavity operations and trials of instrumental delivery[14,15,27–31]. The importance and implications of mid-forceps-associated injury is hotly debated. In the analysis of outcomes for mid-forceps vs. Cesarean delivery, the most important factor is fetal condition at the time of instrumentation[29,30]. With comparable initial fetal condition, outcomes are essentially equal, regardless of mode of delivery. The data are similar for vacuum extraction.

By current ACOG definitions, true mid-pelvic operations by either forceps or the vacuum extractor are increasingly uncommon. They make up less than 1% of all deliveries. If all true mid-pelvic procedures were abandoned and Cesarean delivery performed in these cases, the increase in overall abdominal operative delivery rate would be minimal. It is an unfortunate fact that the ongoing controversy concerning mid-cavity operations generates inappropriate prohibitions against less complex pelvic extractions. Most reviewers, including the authors of this monograph, conclude that not all mid-cavity procedures are inherently hazardous or contraindicated. From an extensive literature review and our clinical experience we believe that a place remains for carefully chosen operations conducted by well-trained surgeons[6–8, 29,30,32].

American obstetric practitioners have faced a rude awaking in terms of the association between intrapartum events and neonatal outcome. Until quite recently, it was widely believed that early diagnosis of fetal compromise or distress would permit appropriate intervention and reduce the likelihood for long-term neurological dysfunction among neonates. Unfortunately, this belief has not been statistically validated[22,23,33,34]. Even extensive reliance on abdominal delivery in complicated cases – such as presumed fetal jeopardy/distress – has not eliminated maternal morbidity nor made a major impact in avoiding either immediate or long-term fetal neurological injury[31,35–37]. Current techniques are best in avoiding fetal *death*. The prevention of neonatal morbidity still eludes us. Thus, even if Cesarean delivery was chosen for all malpresentations, cranial malpositioning or abnormal labors, maternal and some fetal injuries would still occur and not all neonates would prove normal. In this regard, the extensive experience of the group at the National Maternity Hospital in Dublin, Ireland must be acknowledged[38,39]. The active management of labor, emphasizing one-on-one nursing, early amniotomy, aggressive use of oxytocin, and close attention to labor progress, documents the important role of *propulsion* in the clinical management of labor. Nonetheless, modern obstetric practitioners must still face issues of *extraction* in at least a small percentage of cases.

An influence that we imperfectly escape is that of our society and medical culture. When international comparisons are made, it is difficult to ascribe the markedly different rates of operative intervention observed to some inherent variance within human populations or to differences in anatomy[40]. It is quite clear that how we practice is partially due to who we are and the system in which we work. Patterns of practice in induction of labor, technique of oxytocin administration, frequency of use and technique of analgesia/anesthesia, the type of prenatal instruction provided, application of electronic fetal monitoring, and many other factors influence the likelihood of dystocia and resulting management choices.

A critical review of clinical situations associated with an increased incidence of instrumental delivery is helpful in placing these issues and their relationship to operative risks into perspective.

VI.2   ISSUES: RISK ASSESSMENT

2.1   Fetal monitoring

Fetal monitoring, as the term is commonly understood in American practice, usually refers to electronic fetal monitoring (EFM). This technique uses an electronic device to detect and record instantaneous fetal heart rate patterns and uterine contractions on a continuously advancing paper strip. Fetal monitoring during labor can also be accomplished by intermittent auscultation of the fetal heart with a fetoscope or a hand-held portable Doppler device.

In the last 10 years, EFM has become increasingly controversial because of alleged adverse effects and limited efficacy[33,41]. Nevertheless, the majority of major American medical centers still depend on EFM tracings as the principal means of fetal evaluation during labor. There are a number of reasons for this decision, including extensive clinical experience with such devices and the observation that the use of EFM frees nursing personnel for other duties, or permits a single nurse to attend several patients in labor. Given the serious cost restraints of modern medical practice, this trend toward the use of electronic devices to substitute for human observation is likely to be irreversible.

The problems with EFM surround its influence on maternal activity and positioning as well as dilemmas concerning correct interpretation. As commonly practiced, EFM usually restricts the mother to bed and subordinates her positioning and activity to the requirements of a clear signal. The development of various telemetry techniques for EFM may change this in the future.

Most clinicians use EFM as a screening test. Reactive, normal tracings are highly reassuring of fetal well-being. The problem surrounds non-reactive or non-reassuring tracings. These data may or may not reflect fetal hypoxia or acidosis. A correct diagnosis requires further clinical evaluation. Other EFM recordings are frankly ominous. Such tracings include fixed bradycardias, non-reactive tracings with recurrent late decelerations, and patterns of severe, recurrent variable decelerations accompanied by progressive decline in baseline variability[42].

Non-reassuring data require physician interpretation. If less than a fixed bradycardia is present, there is latitude for observation and consideration of additional testing. This might include scalp stimulation (electrode placement, Allis clamp application or digital scalp pinching), fetal acoustic stimulation or performance of scalp sampling, among other evaluation techniques.

If some degree of fetal jeopardy ('distress' or 'non-reassuring tracing', etc.) is diagnosed or suspected, the clinical response is dependent upon the severity of the perceived risk and the dilation and effacement of the mother. As previously discussed, there is a role for vacuum extraction in selected cases of fetal distress when vaginal delivery can proceed more easily and rapidly than a Cesarean operation. Such instances are uncommon, not predictable and require swift, expert management (see Chapter II, Instruments, indications, and issues, Section 2.2.3, Presumed fetal jeopardy/fetal distress).

In the face of acute obstetric difficulty, it is best to follow an established protocol. In our teaching of resident physicians, in cases when fetal well-being is seriously questioned, we emphasize the importance of immediately judging fetal condition by a number of techniques and performing a meticulous vaginal/pelvic examination to determine cervical dilation and effacement, fetal station, and position. The fetopelvic relationship is judged and the vagina carefully palpated for evidence of cord prolapse. The quantity and type of vaginal discharge is noted.

A persistent bradycardia demands prompt delivery if repositioning, discontinuation of oxytocin or other standard interventions fail to result in the resumption of a normal FHR. Mode of delivery is the issue. If fetal distress is suspected or diagnosed, heroic efforts at vaginal delivery are inappropriate and Cesarean delivery is often best. Nonetheless, there should be reasonable restraint in performing abdominal operative procedures for presumed fetal jeopardy when the diagnosis is uncertain or equivocal and/or the vaginal route is not precluded following clinical examination. If the vaginal route proves impossible due to the feto–pelvic relationship or if the clinical situation does not permit delay, Cesarean delivery is promptly performed. The conduct of vaginal trials is discussed in more detail in Chapter II, Instruments, indications, and issues, Section

2.4, Trials of instrumental delivery and Section 3.2, Forceps vs. vacuum extraction operations.

2.2 Dystocia: use of oxytocin

The term dystocia, cephalopelvic disproportion (CPD) or failure to progress (FTP), is used to refer to labor situations in which normal progress does not occur. There is either an arrest or delay in cervical dilation or in the descent of the presenting part (see discussion, Chapter II, Instruments, indications, and issues, Section 3.6, Clinical evaluation of pelvic adequacy).

Many factors influence the progress of labor. Among these are: size of the fetus in relation to the birth canal; adequacy of uterine activity; malpresentation or malpositioning such as cranial deflection; maternal position; coaching; and certain confounding factors such as infection, hydramnios, and the administration of analgesia or anesthesia (especially epidural anesthesia)[43].

Failure to progress is best evaluated by charting cervical dilation and descent of the presenting part, using a standard partogram[15,38,39,43,44]. In general, if normal progress ceases, or if only desultory uterine activity is present, and the pelvis is adequate, the best treatment is a trial of oxytocin uterine stimulation under close observation. In the absence of fetal distress (defined as a normal scalp pH, normal and reactive EFM tracing, or normal auscultatory fetal heart rates in an uncomplicated pregnancy) and with a clinically adequate pelvis, oxytocin stimulation is attempted before resorting to either Cesarean or instrumental delivery.

Judging the point of intervention is not always easy. Both flexibility and humility are necessary in the clinician. Despite our belief in the predictive value of partograms and the accuracy of ultrasonic measurements, the course of labor is neither entirely predictable nor regular. Many clinicians of exceptional competence and vast experience have confidently predicted either uncomplicated labor or inevitable dystocia for a particular case only to be proven completely wrong!

2.3 Problems of anesthesia/analgesia

The use of potent analgesia or anesthesia during labor has always been controversial. Potential adverse effects upon the child, the mother or the course of labor are of concern. While no-one wishes to deny pain relief during delivery, experienced clinicians also recognize that the use of anesthesia can potentially alter labor progress[45–48]. The greatest problem is with epidural anesthesia. Even the recent techniques of constant infusion of low-dose local anesthetics augmented by narcotics cannot provide adequate pain relief without *some* increase in the operative delivery rate. The issue is the cost associated with providing adequate analgesia vs. the benefits to the parturient and her infant from adequate pain relief. Informed obstetric management of the second stage and various changes in modern epidural technique minimize but do not entirely reverse the adverse effects of anesthesia on the course of labor (see discussion, Chapter II, Instruments, indications, and issues, Section 2.4.2, Anesthesia/ analgesia).

2.4   Fetal macrosomia

The excessively large infant represents a recurring and potentially serious obstetric problem[49,50–55]. At the present time, approximately 10% of delivered infants can be expected to weigh 4000 g or greater; and approximately 2.0% are 4500 g or more[51]. Such infants are surprisingly difficult to accurately identify before birth[56–59]. Large babies are more likely to be injured during the birth process than are smaller infants, although the large majority will be delivered easily and atraumatically[54]. The labors of macrosomics are often marked by slow progress, malpresentation or disproportion. Not surprisingly, various fetal injuries and a higher incidence of Cesarean delivery characterize this population.

Major risks for adverse outcome among macrosomic infants occur when efforts at mid-pelvic delivery are accompanied by shoulder dystocia or by unrecognized cranial disproportion. Cesarean delivery reduces the incidence of birth-related damage but does not prevent all birth injuries to large infants.

Simple fetal bulk as reflected in grams of weight is not the only factor in dystocia. Body proportions change as infants become increasingly larger[60]. In general, the trunk and chest increase in size disproportionately to the head as gross body weight increases (Figure VI.1). This predisposes to shoulder dystocia. Other important clinical factors include malpresentation (e.g. occiput posterior or other deflexed postitions), inefficient uterine activity, maternal exhaustion, pelvic architecture, and cervical or soft tissue resistance.

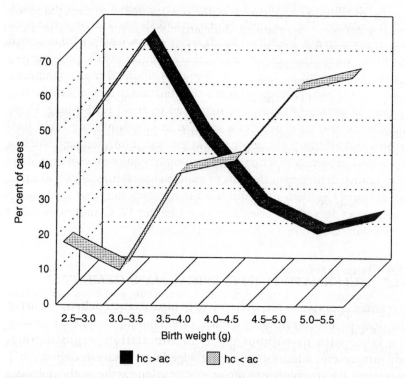

Figure VI.1 Head circumference (hc) to abdominal circumference (ac) plotted against birth weight (n = 137). (Graphic representation of data derived from reference 60)

Avoiding difficult vaginal delivery of macrosomic fetuses is an obvious goal that continues to elude obstetricians. While retrospective studies can identify risk factors for fetal injury, the ability to predict fetopelvic dystocia remains limited, at best[52,53,55]. Many techniques suggested for antepartum evaluation of fetal size are simply unreliable. Physical examination, even by experienced clinicians, is highly inaccurate in estimating fetal weight. Ultrasonic estimates of fetal bulk are similarly problematic with errors of ± 6–10% common[53,55–59]. Similarly, an abnormal labor course may suggest, but does not invariably identify cases of fetopelvic disproportion.

What is important in the fetopelvic relationship is that neither fetus nor pelvis can be evaluated separately from each other. Except in extreme cases, gauging the fit between baby and pelvis is only possible over time by close observation of the classic triad of cervical dilation, station, and cranial position as documented by serial pelvic examinations.

Certain antepartum clinical observations do assist in identifying a high risk population. The diagnosis of maternal diabetes is an important risk factor, prominently identified in all series of macrosomic infants. Past obstetric history is also important. Similarly, a history of the prior birth of a large infant with or without a characteristic birth injury (shoulder dystocia or clavicular fracture) alerts the clinician to a possible repeat.

Several strategies have been suggested to avoid fetal injury. These include elective induction prior to term in cases involving rapid fetal growth and arbitrary ultrasonic weight estimate limits for vaginal trials. None have proven satisfactory. Such proposals require excessive numbers of operative deliveries at the cost of maternal morbidity as well as many unnecessary Cesarean procedures while not avoiding most fetal injury. The correct answer lies elsewhere (see Chapter IV, Complications and birth injuries, Section 2.5, Shoulder dystocia)[53,56].

VI.3 ALTERNATIVES IN CLINICAL MANAGEMENT

A realistic appraisal of the alternatives to instrumental delivery is part of the decision process in every clinical case. Options include continuing the labor with or without oxytocin stimulation, repositioning, encouragement, administration of analgesia or Cesarean delivery[8,61,62]. In general, it is appropriate to prolong labor as long as the mother tolerates the trial, fetal jeopardy/distress is not present, and there is progress in dilation, effacement, and station[13,63,64]. However, if progress ceases following an adequate trial, or if immediate fetal jeopardy/distress is suspected, prompt delivery is indicated.

These are not simple issues. Such concerns in one guise or another have occupied the attention of accoucheurs since the beginning of scientific midwifery. There is continual obstetric debate about what constitutes an adequate trial of labor, how to establish the diagnosis of 'true' fetal jeopardy, and what constitutes the appropriate management of dystocia.

Generally, if progress ceases, close clinical evaluation of the maternal pelvis, size and position of the fetus, and the competence of uterine work is performed. As long as there is no insurmountable difficulty, uterotonics, maternal repositioning, encouragement, judicious use of an oxytocin infusion, low-dose, mixed-agent epidural anesthesia, and extension of the time in labor are used to promote vaginal delivery. This should permit descent of the fetal head. The diagnosis of poor progress in labor is not an immediate indication for either a Cesarean delivery or an instrumental trial if the fetal condition remains good[61,63]. Poor labor progress does, however, require that the clinician reconsider the care provided and establish a new management plan.

In trials of labor, close attention to possible maternal and fetal distress is mandatory. Uterine activity and fetal heart rate are monitored closely[64–66]. Progress is judged by serial pelvic examinations with careful notation of serial cervical dilation, station, and position of the fetal head.

In the absence of disproportion or fetal or maternal distress, coaching, administration of oxytocin, and prolongation of the second stage will either result in spontaneous delivery or a lower station of the fetal head prior to the consideration of an instrumental delivery[8,67–71].

VI.4 ROLE OF VACUUM EXTRACTION

Vacuum extraction is an increasingly popular obstetric procedure in American practice. Use of the extractor complements that of forceps in many services, while in others it essentially replaces them.

There are risks associated with any vaginal delivery[6–8,15]. Both the forceps and the vacuum extractor are imperfect instruments. Even when used properly by well-meaning and skillful clinicians these instruments are capable of inflicting injury to both mother and baby. The cardinal rules of instrumental delivery are simple: neither the vacuum extractor nor the forceps should ever be used without valid indication or by an operator uncertain of the clinical setting or of his or her skill or if true disproportion is suspected[6–8,11].

Despite concerns, vacuum extraction is a safe obstetric procedure[8,11,12,20]. Nonetheless, vacuum operations require careful attention to detail and considerable practice to minimize risk while achieving the benefit of atraumatic vaginal delivery.

REFERENCES

1. Hayes, I. (1831). Editorial comment. In Arnett, N. (ed.) *Elements of Physics or Natural Philosophy, General and Medical, Explained Independently of Technical Mathematics and Containing New Disquisitions and Practical Suggestions*, 2nd edn. (Philadelphia: Carney and Lea)
2. Uhrin, M. (1992). It has been said. *Persp. Biol. Med.*, **35**, 380–1

3. Yancey, M.K., Herposheimer, A., Jordan, G.D., Benson, W.L. and Brady, K. (1991). Maternal and neonatal effects of outlet forceps delivery compared with spontaneous vaginal delivery in term pregnancies. *Obstet. Gynecol.*, **78**, 646–50

4. Newton, E.R. (1988). Complications of operations and procedures for labor and delivery. In Newton, M. and Newton, E.R. (eds.) *Complications of Gynecologic and Obstetric Management*, pp. 315–84. (Philadelphia: WB Saunders)

5. Falco, N.A. and Erickson, E. (1990). Facial nerve palsy in the newborn: incidence and outcome. *Plast. Reconstr. Surg.*, **85**, 1–4

6. Laufe, L.E. and Berkus, M.D. (1992). *Assisted Vaginal Delivery.* (New York: McGraw-Hill Inc.)

7. Dennen, P.C. (1989). *Dennen's Forceps Deliveries*, 3rd edn. (Philadelphia: F.A. Davis Company)

8. O'Grady, J.P. (1988). *Modern Instrumental Delivery.* (Baltimore: Williams & Wilkins)

9. Bishop, E.H., Israel, S.L. and Briscoe, L.C. (1965). Obstetric influences on the premature infant's first year of development. *Obstet. Gynecol.*, **26**, 628–35

10. Blennow, G., Svenningsen, N.W. and Gustafson, B. (1977). Neonatal and prospective follow-up study of infants delivered by vacuum extraction. *Acta Obstet. Gynecol. Scand.*, **56**, 189–94

11. Vacca, A. (1992). *Handbook of Vacuum Extraction in Obstetric Practice.* (London: Edward Arnold)

12. Vacca, A. (1990). The place of the vacuum extractor in modern obstetric practice. *Fet. Med. Rev.*, **119**, 529–42

13. Cohen, W.R. (1977). Influence of the duration of second stage labor on perinatal outcome and puerperal morbidity. *Obstet. Gynecol.*, **49**, 266–8

14. Friedman, E.A., Sachtleben-Murray, M.R., Dahrouge, D. and Negg, R.K. (1985). Long-term effects of labor and delivery and offspring: a matched pair analysis. *Am. J. Obstet. Gynecol.*, **150**, 941–5

15. Friedman, E.A., Acker, D.B. and Sachs, B.P. (1987). *Obstetrical Decision Making*, 2nd edn., pp. 240–1. (Philadelphia: B.C. Decker Inc.)

16. Seidman, D.S., Laor, A., Gale, R. *et al.* (1991). Long-term effects of vacuum and forceps deliveries. *Lancet*, **337**, 1583–5.

17. Bjeer, I. and Dahlin, K. (1974). The long term development of children delivered by vacuum extraction. *Dev. Med. Child Neurol.*, **16**, 378–81

18. Milner, R.D.G. (1975). Neonatal mortality of breech deliveries with and without forceps to the aftercoming head. *Br. J. Obstet. Gynaecol.*, **82**, 783–5

19. McBride, W.G., Black, B.P., Brown, C.J., Dolby, R.M., Murray, A.D. and Thomas, D.B. (1979). Method of delivery and developmental outcome at five years of age. *Med. J. Aust.*, **1**, 301–4

20. Ngan, H.Y.S., Min, P. and Ko, L. (1990). Long-term neurological sequelae following vacuum extractor delivery. *Aust. NZ J. Obstet. Gynaecol.*, **30**, 111–14

21. Bryce, R., Stanley, F. and Blair, E. (1989). The effects of intrapartum care on

the risk of impairment in childhood. In Chalmers, I., Eukin, M. and Keirse, M.J.N.C. (eds.) *Effective Care in Pregnancy and Childhood.* (Oxford: Oxford University Press)

22. Kuban, K.C.K. and Leviton, A. (1994). Cerebral palsy. *N. Engl. J. Med.*, **330**, 188–95

23. Illingsworth, R.S. (1979). Why blame the obstetrician? A review. *Br. Med. J.*, **1**, 797–801

24. Nelson, K.B. and Ellenberg, J.H. (1986). Antecedents of cerebral palsy. *N. Engl. J. Med.*, **315**, 81–6

25. Naeye, R.L. (1992). *Disorders of the Placenta, Fetus, and Neonate: Diagnosis and Clinical Significance.* (St. Louis: Mosby Year Book)

26. Nyirjesy, I. and Pierce, W.E. (1964). Perinatal mortality and maternal morbidity in spontaneous and vaginal deliveries. *Am. J. Obstet. Gynecol.*, **89**, 568–78

27. Friedman, E.A. (1987). Midforceps delivery: No? *Clin. Obstet. Gynecol.*, **30**, 93–105

28. Richardson, D.A., Evans, M.I. and Cibils, L.A. (1983). Midforceps delivery: a critical review. *Am. J. Obstet. Gynecol.*, **145**, 621–32

29. Dierker, L.J.,Jr., Rosen, M.G., Thompson, K., Debanne, S. and Linn, P. (1985). The midforceps: maternal and neonatal outcomes. *Am. J. Obstet. Gynecol.*, **152**, 176–82

30. Dierker, L.J.,Jr., Rosen, M.G., Thompson, K. and Linn, P. (1986). Midforceps deliveries: long-term outcome of infants. *Am. J. Obstet. Gynecol.*, **154**, 764–8

31. Verma, U.L. (1990). A critical analysis of the long-term sequelae of midcavity forceps delivery. In Tejani, N. (ed.) *Obstetrical Events and Developmental Sequelae*, 2nd edn., pp. 161–79. (Boca Raton: CRC Press Inc.)

32. deVilliers, V.P. (1991). Obstetric forceps after a failed ventouse application. *S. Afr. Med. J.*, **80**, 301

33. Freeman, R. (1990). Intrapartum fetal monitoring – a disappointing story. *N. Engl. J. Med.*, **322**, 624–6

34. Naeye, R.L. and Peters, E.C. (1987). Antenatal hypoxia and low IQ values. *Am. J. Dis. Child.*, **141**, 50–4

35. Opit, L.G. and Selwood, T.S. (1979). Cesarean section rates in Australia: a population-based audit. *Med. J. Aust.*, **2**, 706–9

36. Sunshine, P. (1989). Epidemiology of perinatal asphyxia. In Stevenson, D.K. and Sunshine, P. (eds.) *Fetal and Neonatal Brain Injury: Mechanisms, Management, and the Risks of Practice*, pp. 2–10. (Philadelphia: B.C. Decker)

37. Cattamanchi, G.R., Tamaskar, V., Egel, R.T., Singh, R.S., Yrapsis, N.S., Patel, V. and Rathi, M. (1981). Intrauterine quadraplegia associated with breech presentation and hyperextension of the fetal head: a case report. *Am. J. Obstet. Gynecol.*, **140**, 831–3

38. O'Driscoll, K., Foley, M. and MacDonald, D. (1984). Active management of

labor as an alternative to cesarean section for dystocia. *Obstet. Gynecol.*, **63**, 485–90

39. O'Driscoll, K., Meagher, D. and Boylan, P. (1993). *Active Management of Labor*, 3rd edn. (Aylesbury: Mosby Yearbook Europe Limited)

40. Lomas, J. and Eukin, M. (1989). Variations in operative delivery rates. In Chalmers, I., Eukin, M. and Kierse, M.J.N.C. (eds.) *Effective Care in Pregnancy and Childbirth*, pp. 1182–95. (Oxford: Oxford University Press)

41. Banta, H. and Thacker, S. (1979). Assessing the costs and benefits of electronic fetal monitoring. *Obstet. Gynecol. Surv.*, **34**, 627–42

42. Gaziano, E.P., Freeman, D.W. and Bendel, R.P. (1980). FHR variability and other heart rate observations during second stage labor. *Obstet. Gynecol.*, **56**, 42–7

43. Gee, H. and Oláh, K.S. (1993). Failure to progress in labour. In Studd, J. (ed.) *Progress in Obstetrics and Gynaecology*, vol. 10, pp. 159–82. (Edinburgh: Churchill-Livingstone)

44. Studd, J. (1973). Partograms and nomograms of cervical dilatation in management of primigravid labour. *Br. Med. J.*, **4**, 451–5

45. Thorp, J.A., Parisi, V.M., Boylan, P.C. and Johnston, D.A. (1989). The effect of continuous epidural analgesia on cesarean section for dystocia in nulliparous women. *Am. J. Obstet. Gynecol.*, **161**, 670–5

46. Chestnut, D.H. (1991). Epidural anesthesia and instrumental vaginal delivery. *J. Anesthesiol.*, **74**, 805–8

47. Youngstrom, P. and O'Grady, J.P. (1990). Must epidurals always imply instrumental delivery? *Contemp. Ob./Gyn.*, **35**, 19–27

48. Chestnut, D.H., McGrath, J.M., Vincent, R.D., Jr., Penning, D.H., Choi, W.W., Bates, J.N. and McFarlane, C. (1994). Does early administration of epidural anesthesia affect obstetric outcome in nulliparous women who are receiving intravenous oxytocin? *Anesthesiology*, **80**, 1193–200

49. Levine, M.G., Holroyde, J. and Woods, J.R. (1984). Birth trauma: incidence and predisposing factors. *Obstet. Gynecol.*, **63**, 792–5

50. Mondanlou, H.D., Komatsu, G., Dorchester, W., Freeman, R.K. and Bosu, S.K. (1982). Large-for-gestational-age neonates: anthropometric reasons for shoulder dystocia. *Obstet. Gynecol.*, **60**, 417–23

51. Boyd, M.E., Usher, R.H. and McLean, F.H. (1983). Fetal macrosomia: prediction, risks, proposed management. *Obstet. Gynecol.*, **61**, 715–22

52. O'Leary, J.A. (1992). *Shoulder Dystocia and Birth Injury*. (New York: McGraw-Hill Inc.)

53. Sandmire, H.F. and O'Hallin, T.J. (1988). Shoulder dystocia: its incidence and associated risk factors. *Int. Gynecol. Obstet.*, **26**, 65–73

54. Menticoglou, S.M., Manning, F.A., Morrison, I. and Harman, C.R. (1992). Must macrosomic fetuses be delivered by a Cesarean section? A review of outcome for 786 babies ≥ 4500 g. *Aust. NZ J. Obstet. Gynaecol.*, **32**, 100–3

55. Gross, T.L., Sokol, R.J., Williams, T. and Thomson, K. (1987). Shoulder dystocia: a fetal-physician risk. *Am. J. Obstet. Gynecol.*, **156**, 1408–18

56. Sandmire, H.F. (1993). Whither ultrasonic prediction of fetal macrosomia. *Obstet. Gynecol.*, **82**, 860–2

57. Sabagha, R.E., Minoque. J., Tamura, R.K. and Hungerford, S.A. (1989). Estimation of birth weight by use of ultrasonic formulas targeted to large-appropriate, and small-for-gestational-age fetuses. *Am. J. Obstet. Gynecol.*, **160**, 854–62

58. Chervenak, J.L., Divon, M.Y., Hirsch, J., Girz, B.A. and Langer, O. (1989). Macrosomia in the post date pregnancy: is routine ultrasonographic screening indicated? *Am. J. Obstet. Gynecol.*, **161**, 753–6

59. Hirata, G.I., Medearis, A.L., Horenstein, J., Bear, M.B. and Platt, L.D. (1990). Ultrasonographic estimation of fetal weight in the clinically macrosomic fetus. *Am. J. Obstet. Gynecol.*, **162**, 238–42

60. Seigworth, G.R. (1966). Shoulder dystocia: review of 5 years' experience. *Obstet. Gynecol.*, **28**, 764–7

61. Cohen, W. (1983). The pelvic division of labor. In Cohen, W.R. and Friedman, E.A. (eds.) *Management of Labor*, pp. 41–64. (Baltimore: University Park Press)

62. Compton, A.A. (1990). Avoiding difficult vaginal deliveries. In Dilts, P.V. and Sciarra, J.J. (eds.) *Gynecology and Obstetrics*, vol. 2, 74, pp. 1–8. (Philadelphia: JB Lippincott Company)

63. Bottoms, S.F., Hirsch, V.J. and Sokol, R.J. (1987). Medical management of arrest disorders of labor: a current overview. *Am. J. Obstet. Gynecol.*, **156**, 935–9

64. American College of Obstetricians and Gynecologists (1989). *Dystocia.* Technical Bulletin No. 137. (Washington, DC: American College of Obstetricians and Gynecologists)

65. Hauth, J.C., Hankins, G.D., Gilstrap, L.C. 3rd, Strickland, D.M. and Vance, P. (1986). Uterine contraction pressures with oxytocin induction/augmentation. *Obstet. Gynecol.*, **68**, 305–9

66. Neuhoff, D., Burks, M.S. and Porreco, R.P. (1989). Cesarean birth for failed progression in labor. *Obstet. Gynecol.*, **73**, 915–20

67. Studd, J.W., Crawford, J.S., Duignan, N.M., Rowbotham, C.J. and Hughes, A.O. (1980). The effect of lumbar epidural analgesia on the rate of cervical dilatation and the outcome of labour of spontaneous onset. *Br. J. Obstet. Gynaecol.*, **87**, 1015–21

68. Drife, J.O. (1983). Kielland or Caesar? *Br. Med. J.*, **287**, 309–10

69. Crawford, J.S. (1983). The stages and phases of labour: an outworn nomenclature that invites hazard. *Lancet*, **ii**, 271–2

70. Saunders, N.J., Spiby, H., Gilbert, L., Fraser, R.B., Hall, J.M., Mutton, P.M., Jackson, A. and Edmonds, D.K. (1989). Oxytocin infusion during second stage of labour in primiparous women using epidural analgesia: a randomised double bind placebo controlled study. *Br. Med. J.*, **299**, 1423–6

71. Garbaciak, J.A. (1990). Labor and delivery: anesthesia, induction of labor, malpresentation, and operative delivery. *Curr. Opin. Obstet. Gynecol.*, **2**, 773–9

Index

Page numbers in **bold type** refer to figures, and those in *italics* to tables.

Knowledge is of two kinds. We know a subject ourselves, or we know where we can find information upon it.

Samuel Johnson
18 April 1775

The Oxford Dictionary of Quotations, (1979), 3rd edn., p. 276.
(Oxford: Oxford University Press)